Asthma Care in the Community

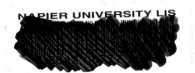

Asthma Care in the Community

JILL WALDRON RN, BSc (Hons)
Respiratory Specialist Nurse
Cornwall & Isles of Scilly Primary Care Trust

BICENTENNIAL
1807
WILEY
2007
BICENTENNIAL

John Wiley & Sons, Ltd

Copyright © 2007   John Wiley & Sons, Ltd
The Atrium, Southern Gate, Chichester,
West Sussex PO19 8SQ, England
Telephone   (+44) 1243 779777

E-mail (for orders and customer service enquiries): cs-books@wiley.co.uk
Visit our Home Page on www.wiley.com

Other Wiley Editorial Offices

John Wiley & Sons Inc., 111 River Street, Hoboken, NJ 07030, USA

Jossey-Bass, 989 Market Street, San Francisco, CA 94103-1741, USA

Wiley-VCH Verlag GmbH, Boschstr. 12, D-69469 Weinheim, Germany

John Wiley & Sons Australia Ltd, 42 McDougall Street, Milton, Queensland 4064, Australia

John Wiley & Sons (Asia) Pte Ltd, 2 Clementi Loop #02-01, Jin Xing Distripark, Singapore 129809

John Wiley & Sons Canada Ltd, 6045 Freemont Blvd, Mississauga, ONT, L5R 4J3, Canada

Wiley also publishes its books in a variety of electronic formats. Some content that appears in print may
not be available in electronic books.

Anniversary Logo Design: Richard J. Pacifico

Library of Congress Cataloging-in-Publication Data

Waldron, Jill.
  Asthma care in the community / Jill Waldron.
    p. ; cm.
  Includes bibliographical references.
  ISBN 978-0-470-03000-4 (pbk. : alk. paper)
  1. Asthma.   2. Asthma–Treatment.   I. Title.
  [DNLM: 1. Asthma–nursing.   2. Holistic Nursing–methods.   3. Patient Care
  Management–methods.
  WY 163 W167a 2007]
  RC591.W25 2007

  616.2'38–dc22

                                                            2007014620

British Library Cataloguing in Publication Data
A catalogue record for this book is available from the British Library

ISBN: 978-0-470-03000-4

Typeset by Aptara, Inc., Delhi, India.
Printed and bound in Great Britain by TJ International Ltd, Padstow, Cornwall.
This book is printed on acid-free paper responsibly manufactured from sustainable forestry in which at
least two trees are planted for each one used for paper production.

Contents

Preface

Asthma is a common, chronic condition affecting all age groups. It is sometimes easy to forget that, despite being so common, it is still a disease with high levels of morbidity and unacceptable rates of mortality.

The pathology and management of asthma can be very complex. However, to the patient more often than not, it is the simple aspects of asthma management that can really make a difference to their day-to-day life. This book has been written, therefore, with the aim of guiding the practitioner through the asthma patient journey in a logical, sequential approach. It addresses the more complex issues but also emphasizes the 'back to basics' approach.

As health professionals we are constantly aiming to improve our skills and knowledge. Although written primarily for nurses, clinicians in other fields of healthcare should find the book a useful tool towards meeting some of those aims. By working with a multidisciplinary approach, the holistic needs of people with asthma can be addressed. The author is an experienced respiratory specialist nurse, with over ten years' experience of working with asthma patients and their families in the community. I hope you will find it an enjoyable and informative read.

Acknowledgements

I would like to thank my husband and family for their support in writing this book. The finished product has come about as a result of their tolerance, and their help with proofreading.

I would also like to thank my colleague Deirdre Denn for her valuable contributions and ideas.

Introduction

Asthma is a variable condition which may manifest itself in many different ways. It often leads to impaired quality of life and can have an impact on family relationships. Although more common in children, asthma can occur at any age, and this book aims to look at the evidence-based management of this diverse patient group, from a community perspective.

The information in this book is based on the British Thoracic Society Guidelines (BTS) [1]. It starts with a brief overview of epidemiology, anatomy and physiology and an introduction to asthma medications. We then follow the patient journey from a diagnosis of asthma to the management and care of this chronic condition. Each chapter addresses the different issues involved in asthma management but can be used in a 'stand alone' format to approach specific issues.

The Glossary at the end of the book explains terminology and abbreviations and there is a section of useful addresses. Case studies and vignettes have been used throughout the text to illustrate certain points.

The management of asthma is being delegated more and more to nurses working in different areas of healthcare. It is important that their skills and knowledge are up to date. I hope this book will go some way to meeting these needs.

REFERENCE

1. British Thoracic Society/Scottish Intercollegiate Guidelines Network (2005) *British Guideline on the Management of Asthma*, Revised edition. Available at www.brit-thoracic.org.uk.

1   The Epidemiology of Asthma

Key points:

- Asthma is one of the most common chronic diseases, affecting all age groups.
- It is currently estimated that 300 million people in the world have a diagnosis of asthma.
- In the UK, 5.2 million people currently receive treatment for asthma.
- In the UK, one in ten children have a diagnosis of asthma.
- The incidence of asthma is highest in affluent English-speaking countries.
- Asthma mortality is falling but the majority of asthma deaths are preventable.
- In 2005, 1136 people died as a result of asthma.
- Asthma costs the NHS £889 million a year.
- The total cost of asthma to the UK economy is £2.3 billion a year when you take into account sickness benefits and lost production.

INTRODUCTION

Asthma is one of the most common chronic diseases affecting all age groups, and is particularly prevalent in children. Despite a lot of research, it is still not known why some people get asthma and some don't. We do know that it is more common in people who have a family history of asthma or related atopic conditions such as eczema or allergic rhinitis, and also that people who have these allergic-type diseases themselves are more likely to suffer from asthma.

INCIDENCE AND PREVALENCE

The incidence of a condition refers to the number of new cases that arise during a specified period of time. Prevalence describes the proportion of people who have that condition, and may be measured at a single point in time, over a defined period of time or over an individual's entire lifetime.

It has been estimated that around 300 million people in the world currently have asthma, with large variations in prevalence in different regions. The condition is much more prevalent in childhood, and it is thought that at least one in ten children currently have a diagnosis of asthma in the UK. It is also more common in boys than in girls during childhood, but this difference evens out as children approach adolescence and then it becomes more common in girls.

True figures about the prevalence of asthma are very difficult to ascertain due to methodological difficulties in obtaining this sort of data. There are large variations in classification, and inconsistent methods of interpreting symptoms in different countries. Diagnostic procedures are not consistent as there is no specific diagnostic tool that can be used to identify asthma. Most of the data therefore is derived from written questionnaires which have used the occurrence of self-reported wheeze as being the most important symptom for identifying asthma. The two main studies to report on asthma prevalence used this format and asked specifically about self-reported wheeze in the previous 12 months.

The International Study of Asthma and Allergies in Childhood (ISAAC), in its Phase 1 Study [1], investigated symptom prevalence in children in the 13–14 year age group and found that prevalence varied between 6 and 32 %. Prevalence was lowest in India, Eastern Europe, China and the former Soviet Union, and highest in the affluent English-speaking countries. The other study, the European Community Respiratory Health Survey (ECRHS) [2] concentrated on the 20–44 year age group, and found an overall prevalence of 6.9 %, with prevalence being highest in Australia, New Zealand, the United States and the UK, and lowest in parts of Spain, Germany, Italy and India.

In its Phase 111 study [3], ISAAC found that the prevalence of asthma, allergic rhinoconjunctivitis and eczema is continuing to increase in the younger age group children, that is children aged 6–7 years, but decreasing in those children in the higher age group, that is children in the 13–14 year age range.

Despite general acceptance of this method of collecting information, it should be recognized that there are a number of limitations in the interpretation of such data. It can not be taken for granted that self-reported wheeze is diagnostic of asthma, as wheeze can be a symptom of many respiratory diseases. Many children, for example, have wheezing episodes during infancy that never become asthma. Similarly, older children and adults may suffer from respiratory infections which cause wheezing, but which disappear after treatment.

In the UK in 2003, the General Medical Services Contract for General Practitioners was introduced [4]. One of the components of the Contract is the Quality and Outcomes Framework (QOF), which was developed to try to improve the quality of care for a number of long-term conditions, including asthma. The QOF identifies certain service indicators for each condition and the practice is financially rewarded if these indicators are achieved. One of the indicators for asthma is that the practice can produce a register of asthma patients. Although at present this data has not been validated for epidemiological purposes, it is thought that in the future it may well provide a valuable and reliable source of information about asthma prevalence in the UK.

Until there is considerable improvement and agreement in diagnostic criteria between countries, however, the self-reported questionnaire continues to be the mainstay of obtaining data about the prevalence of asthma worldwide.

PREVALENCE OF ASTHMA IN THE UK

In the UK, it is estimated that 5.2 million people currently receive treatment for asthma, 1.1 million of these are children under the age of 16 [5]. In its recently updated statistics report, the British Thoracic Society [6] state that in England, about 4 % of the population report wheezing in the past year. Recent reports from the QOF data suggest that the number of patients currently being treated for asthma range from 3.2 to 7.4 % across England [7]. This variation is thought to reflect differences in age groups and socio-economic factors.

MORTALITY

Fortunately, deaths from asthma are not common and the death rate is steadily falling, although not as fast as one would hope, given that there are much more effective treatment strategies available now than there were in the past. Over the last 40–50 years, mortality from asthma has declined; however, there have been several, short-lived, and largely unexplained, increases in asthma mortality. For example in the mid 1960s there appeared to be an increase in the numbers of asthma deaths reported, which was thought to be related to certain medication usage, as will be discussed later in this chapter. Similarly in the late 1980s and early 1990s there was a sharp rise in numbers of asthma deaths, but it has been suggested that changes in diagnostic practices, especially in differentiating between COPD and asthma, may explain this event. Up until around the mid 1990s, about 2000 people died every year from asthma in the UK. However, since then, there has been a slow but steady decrease as shown in Figure 1.1. In 2005, 1136 people died as a result of asthma.

The sad fact about asthma deaths is that a large proportion of them should never have happened. In 1982, the then British Thoracic Association published a study looking at asthma deaths in England and found that 86 % of these deaths may have been preventable by better management [8]. The report concluded that patients needed more rigorous drug treatment and better follow-up. It would be reasonable to expect that things have improved since then; however, subsequent studies are still showing serious shortcomings in asthma management and, unfortunately, unnecessary deaths [9–11]. These studies highlighted under-treatment with inhaled steroids and inadequate routine monitoring of patients.

A number of other contributing factors to asthma deaths were also identified in these studies which are much more difficult to deal with. These included patient behaviour and circumstances. In all the studies, the majority of patients who died from asthma were shown to have adverse psychosocial factors such as depression, psychosis, stress or poor living conditions. It was also found that many patients who died from asthma delayed calling for medical help in the final, fatal attack. Poor concordance with preventer medication and over-reliance on reliever inhalers have also been shown to contribute to asthma deaths.

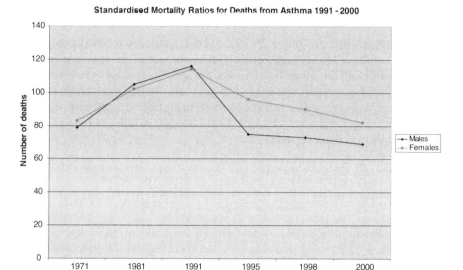

Figure 1.1. Standardized mortality ratio for asthma deaths from 1991 to 2000.
Source of data: National Statistics Office: Mortality Statistics by Cause. Series DH2 no.32.

Over the last 30–40 years there has been a great debate as to whether the use of short-acting B2 agonists has contributed to asthma deaths. In the mid 1960s, for example, there was a sharp rise and subsequent fall in asthma deaths in several countries, including the United Kingdom, which was linked to the introduction of isoprenaline, a nonselective B agonist drug. The death rate fell when the drug was subsequently withdrawn. In New Zealand in the 1970s, an increase in asthma deaths corresponded to an increase in prescriptions for another B2 agonist, fenoterol.

Three recent studies [12–14] found that there was high usage of short-acting bronchodilators among patients who died from asthma, but the authors could not conclude whether the drugs actually contributed to these deaths. It has been suggested that patients with severe disease would naturally be using more short-acting bronchodilators, and that it was the severity of the disease rather than the drugs that actually caused the deaths.

In 2006, the results of a large American study were published investigating asthma deaths in relation to the use of long-acting B2 agonists. This study concluded that there were more asthma deaths in the group of patients using a long-acting B2 agonist than in the placebo group [15]. However, the majority of the patients who died were not using an inhaled steroid and were from a more disadvantaged social background. Similarly, a meta-analysis of studies looking at long-acting B2 agonist use and asthma severity found that those patients using these drugs had a higher hospital admission rate and episodes of life-threatening asthma [16]. However, there has been some debate as to the interpretation of the data of this particular study. In contrast to both these studies, researchers in the UK found that there was no connection between asthma deaths and the use of long-acting B2 agonists [17]. The Commission on Human Medicines has now recommended that further, reliable research is conducted into this issue. (See Chapters 5 and 7 for current advice on the use of long-acting B2 agonist drugs.)

Asthma mortality is now falling by about 6 % each year in England and Wales.

THE ECONOMIC AND SOCIAL BURDEN OF ASTHMA

It is estimated that asthma is costing the National Health Service (NHS) over £889 million a year [5]. The majority of this cost is taken up by prescriptions, closely followed by GP consultations and hospital admissions. However, other factors also have to be taken into account such as lost productivity, and social security benefits because of sickness and absence from work. The total cost is thought to be more in the region of £2.3 billion a year when these other factors are taken into account.

SUMMARY

Asthma is a common, chronic condition affecting all age groups, but with the highest prevalence in children. Accurate data is difficult to obtain due to methodological difficulties in collecting the information. It is important, however, to try to gain reliable information about the prevalence of asthma in order to develop services, and target resources effectively.

Mortality from asthma is fortunately relatively rare, but given that there are very effective treatments available for asthma, the death rate is unacceptable. Studies have shown that the majority of asthma deaths may have been preventable by better management and follow-up. We should also be looking for ways of reaching patients who are psychologically, or socially disadvantaged, as this group of people has been shown to be more likely to suffer fatal or near fatal attacks of asthma.

REFERENCES

1. Kaur, B., Anderson, H.R., Austin, J. *et al.* (1998) Prevalence of asthma symptoms, diagnosis, and treatment in 12–14 year old children across Great Britain (international study of asthma and allergies in childhood, ISAAC UK). *British Medical Journal*, **316**, 118–24.
2. European Community Respiratory Health Survey (1996) Variation in the prevalence of respiratory symptoms, self-reported asthma attacks, and use of asthma medication in the European Community Respiratory Health Survey (ECRHS). *European Respiratory Journal*, **9**, 698–5.
3. Innes Asher, M., Montefort, S., Bjorksten, B. *et al.* (2006) Worldwide time trends in the prevalence of symptoms of asthma, allergic rhinoconjunctivitis, and eczema in childhood: ISAAC Phases One and Three repeat multicountry cross-sectional surveys. *The Lancet*, **368**, 733–43.

4. Department of Health (2003) *Quality and Outcomes Framework*. www.dh.gov.uk.
5. Asthma UK (2004) *Where Do We Stand. Asthma in the UK Today*. www.asthma.org.uk.
6. British Thoracic Society (2006) *The Burden of Lung Disease*, 2nd edn. A Statistics Report from the British Thoracic Society. www.brit-thoracic.org.uk.
7. Lung & Asthma Information Agency (2006) Estimating the prevalence of asthma: QOF v Health Survey for England. www.laia.ac.uk/QOF.htm.
8. British Thoracic Association (1982) Deaths from Asthma in Two Regions of England. *British Medical Journal*, **285**, 1251–5.
9. Bucknall, C.E., Slack, R., Godley, C.C. *et al.* (1999) Scottish confidential inquiry into asthma deaths (SCIAD), 1994–1996. *Thorax*, **54** (11), 978–84.
10. Burr, M.L., Davies, B.H., Hoare, A. *et al.* (1999) A confidential inquiry into asthma deaths in Wales. *Thorax*, **54** (11), 985–9.
11. Sturdy, P.M., Butland, B.K., Anderson, H.R. *et al.* on behalf of the National Asthma Campaign Mortality and Severe Morbidity Group (2005) Deaths certified as asthma and use of medical services: a national case-control study. *Thorax*, **60**, 909–15.
12. Anderson, H.R., Ayres, J.G., Sturdy, P.M. *et al.* (2005) Bronchodilator treatment and deaths from asthma: case-control study. *British Medical Journal*, **330**, 117–23.
13. Lanes, S.F., Birman, B., Raiford, D. and Walker, A.M. (1997) International trends in sales of inhaled fenoterol, all inhaled beta-agonists, and asthma mortality, 1970–1992. *Journal of Clinical Epidemiology*, **50** (3), 321–8.
14. Garrett, J.E., Lanes, S.F., Kolbe, J. and Rea, H.H. (1996) Risk of severe life threatening asthma and beta agonist type: an example of confounding by severity. *Thorax*, **51** (11), 1093–9.
15. Nelson, H.S., Weiss, S.T., Bleeker, E.R. *et al.* (2006) The salmeterol multicenter asthma research trial. A comparison of usual pharmacotherapy for asthma or usual pharmacotherapy plus salmeterol. *Chest*, **129**, 15–26.
16. Salpeter, S.R., Buckley, N.S., Ormiston, T.M. and Salpeter, E.E. (2006) Meta-analysis: Effect of long-acting B-agonists on severe asthma exacerbations and asthma-related deaths. *Annals of Internal Medicine*, **144** (Iss 12).
17. Ross Anderson, H., Ayres, J.G., Sturdy, P.M. *et al.* (2005) Bronchodilator treatment and deaths from asthma: case-control study. *British Medical Journal*, **330**, 117.

2 The Respiratory System

INTRODUCTION

Respiration is essential to human life. The main function of the respiratory system is to maintain the balance of oxygen and carbon dioxide in the lungs and tissues. The word respiration is applied to two processes:

- Breathing or external respiration, in which oxygen is taken from the inhaled air and carbon dioxide is breathed out
- Internal or cellular respiration, in which oxygen diffuses into the blood in order to supply the body cells with a sufficient supply of oxygen essential for their cellular metabolism. The carbon dioxide which is generated from this process must then be eliminated.

The respiratory system refers collectively to the lungs, upper and lower respiratory tract and the thoracic cavity, and can be conveniently divided into the upper and lower respiratory tracts. It has a number of different components, but before going on to describe these components, it is important to understand the structure and function of the different layers of cells that make up the respiratory system. Within the respiratory system a variety of respiratory surfaces have been developed in order to increase the surface area in which the exchange of oxygen and carbon dioxide can occur. These cells have certain common features, but there are slight variations in different areas, which will be explained under their respective headings.

THE STRUCTURE OF THE AIRWAYS

The airways consist of respiratory, ciliated epithelium, which is a layer of cells, resting on the basement membrane. The basement membrane separates the epithelium from the submucosa. In the trachea and bronchi the cells are tall and called columnar epithelium. In the smaller bronchioles the cells are short and called cuboidal epithelium.

Beneath the basement membrane lies the lamina propria. This is a layer of connective tissue containing a network of nerve fibres and capillaries supplying the lung. Together with the epithelium it forms the mucosa. Under the lamina propria lies the submucosa, containing mucus-secreting glands, and bronchial smooth muscle.

This muscle consists of two sets of muscle fibres which wind around the bronchi and bronchioles in a double spiral. It looks a bit like a Greek sandal strap winding around the ankle and leg. The bronchial smooth muscle is able to relax and constrict, depending on contributing factors which will be discussed further on in this chapter. Figure 2.1 shows a cross section of a bronchus.

Mucous glands and goblet cells situated in the epithelium secrete a sticky mucus which helps to keep the lining of the airways moist and also traps small particles of inhaled dust, or other foreign matter. These particles are then taken up by cilia which

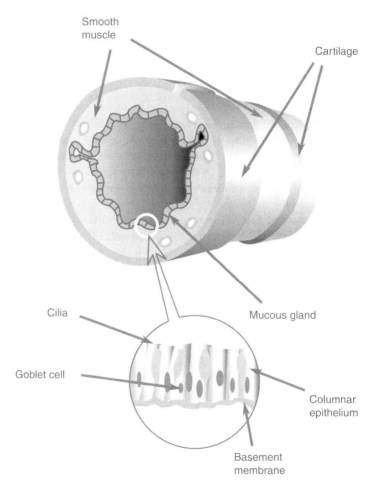

Figure 2.1. Cross section of a bronchus.

are tiny hairs that constantly beat with a whip-like action. Their function is to move mucus and any particles that may be trapped in the mucus, upwards to the pharynx. The mucous glands, goblet cells and cilia are collectively known as the mucociliary system and are the respiratory system's first line of defence against inhaled foreign substances.

These structures are illustrated in Figure 2.1.

THE UPPER RESPIRATORY TRACT

The upper respiratory tract consists of:

- the nose
- the mouth
- the pharynx
- the larynx

THE NOSE

The nose consists of two parts, the external nose which is very obviously visible on the face, and the internal nose. The internal nose contains the nasal cavities, the main functions of which are smelling and breathing. The lower two-thirds of the nasal cavity is lined with ciliated columnar epithelium, also known as respiratory epithelium, and mucous membrane. The cilia prevent inhaled particles from reaching the lungs and help to propel secretions to the pharynx, where they can either be coughed up or swallowed. The mucous membrane helps to keep the nasal cavities moist and has a very rich blood supply, warming inspired air before it reaches the lungs. The main function of this part of the nose therefore is to warm, moisten and filter inspired air.

THE PHARYNX

The pharynx extends from the base of the skull until it joins with the trachea at the front and the oesophagus at the back. It is divided into three parts: the nasopharynx, the oropharynx and the laryngopharynx. The nasopharynx lies above the soft palate which cuts it off from the oropharynx during swallowing. The oropharynx and laryngopharynx are lined with stratified squamous epithelium and also contain many salivary glands which help to keep the structures moist.

THE LARYNX

The larynx is a cartilaginous structure with three main functions. These are:

- voice production
- to protect the trachea and bronchi during swallowing
- to allow the passage of air in and out of the lungs

The upper end of the larynx is continuous with the oropharynx, and is lined with stratified epithelium. The bottom end, which is lined with ciliated epithelium, joins on to the trachea, where the lower respiratory tract begins. At the front of the larynx is a flap of cartilage called the epiglottis. At rest the epiglottis is upright allowing air to pass through the larynx into the lungs. During swallowing, the epiglottis folds back to cover the entrance to the larynx, preventing food or drink from entering the trachea.

Because this book is about asthma and the respiratory system, the emphasis is on the structures involved in breathing. However, it should be remembered that the upper respiratory tract also plays a part in the way we enjoy our food as it contains the organs responsible for taste, smell, chewing and swallowing.

LOWER RESPIRATORY TRACT

The lower respiratory tract consists of:

- the trachea
- the right and left main bronchus
- the smaller bronchi
- the bronchioles
- the lungs

These structures are illustrated in Figure 2.2

THE TRACHEA

The trachea in adults is usually about 10 cm long and 2.5 cm in diameter. It extends from the larynx to the middle of the thorax where it divides into the two primary bronchi. It is a muscular tube supported by C-shaped rings of cartilage which help to protect it and prevent it from collapsing. The gap in the rings of cartilage lies at the back where the trachea is in contact with the oesophagus.

The wall of the trachea is made up of involuntary muscle and fibrous tissue, and lined with ciliated columnar epithelium with a thick basement membrane. The lamina propria is loose and highly vascular. The loose submucosa contains mucus producing glands.

BRONCHI

The trachea divides into the right and left main bronchus (two = bronchi), leading into each lung. The left main bronchus is longer and slightly more horizontal than the right main bronchus, to take account of the position of the heart. This is the reason why an inhaled foreign body invariably ends up in the right main bronchus, because it is straighter and more vertical, making it an easier passage for objects such as nuts and beads.

The respiratory tract

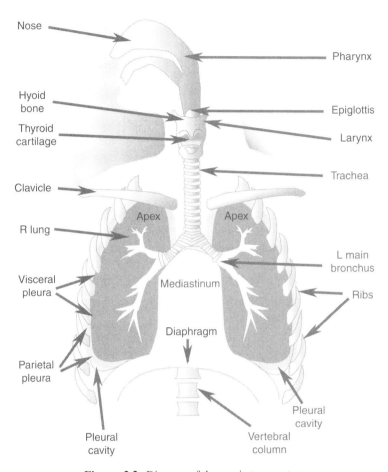

Figure 2.2. Diagram of the respiratory system.

The structure of the bronchi is similar to the trachea, but the cartilage is less regular and the epithelium is shorter and contains fewer goblet cells. The lamina propria is denser and contains mast cells, which play an important part in the inflammatory process. It is separated from the submucosa by a layer of smooth muscle.

The bronchi divide into secondary, or lobar bronchi, and again into tertiary, or segmental bronchi. This process continues with the bronchi becoming smaller at each division until they eventually become bronchioles. As the bronchi get smaller, the cartilage starts to disappear, the lamina propria becomes thinner and more elastic and the smooth muscle layer plays a more prominent part in supporting the airways.

BRONCHIOLES

Eventually the whole thing looks like an upside down tree, with the bronchioles forming the twigs at the end of the branches. These tiny bronchioles are lined with cuboidal epithelium and have no cartilage. The walls of the bronchioles are made up of smooth muscle and fibrous and elastic tissue which helps to support them and keep them patent. The patency of the airways is also aided by air pressure within the bronchioles.

The smallest bronchioles, called respiratory bronchioles, consist of just a single layer of flattened epithelial cells surrounded by smooth muscle. There are no goblet cells, and alveoli are present in the airway walls, allowing some gaseous exchange to take place. Finally, the bronchioles immediately next to the alveoli are called terminal bronchioles which lead into the acinus.

THE ACINUS

This part of the respiratory system is involved with gas exchange, and is also known as the blood–air interface. Gas exchange is the passage of oxygen from the lungs to the bloodstream and the passage of carbon dioxide from the bloodstream to the lungs. The acinus consists of:

• the respiratory bronchioles, which lead into the alveolar ducts
• the alveolar ducts which open into the alveoli

The tiny respiratory bronchioles eventually become alveolar ducts which terminate in groups of thin-walled sacs called alveoli (singular, alveolus) where gas exchange takes place. Alveolar ducts are tiny passages made up of rings of smooth muscle with collagen and elastic fibres. They also have alveoli present in their walls.

THE ALVEOLI

The respiratory tract terminates with the gas exchanging units, the alveoli. They are about 0.1–0.2 mm in diameter, and are surrounded by a large network of capillaries. There are about 200–400 million alveoli in each lung, which is equivalent to the surface area of two tennis courts! This provides a huge area for gas exchange to take place. The alveoli have very thin walls, lined with type I and type II pneumocytes which sit on the basement membrane. Type I pneumocytes make up 40 % of the cells present in the alveoli. They are very thin and aid gas exchange. Type II pneumocytes make up the other 60 % of cells and secrete surfactant which helps to prevent alveolar collapse by reducing the surface tension of the alveolar lining fluid. They also prevent transudation of fluid into the alveoli.

Figure 2.3 illustrates the bronchial tree leading into the alveoli.

The lungs and bronchial tree

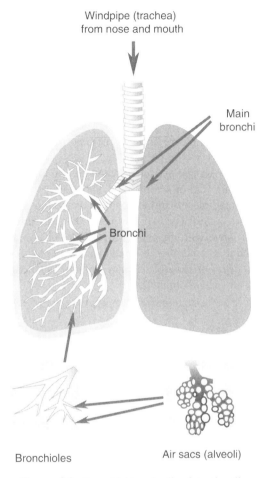

Windpipe (trachea)
from nose and mouth

Main
bronchi

Bronchi

Bronchioles

Air sacs (alveoli)

Figure 2.3. Bronchial tree leading into alveoli.

THE LUNGS

The lungs are spongy, cone-shaped structures and are divided by the mediastinum. They contain the airways, blood vessels, lymph nodes, nerves and supportive connective tissue. The left lung has two lobes and is slightly smaller than the right lung which has three lobes. The base of the lungs rests on the diaphragm, and the top, which is called the apex, starts at the root of the neck.

The lung tissue contains elastic fibres and collagen which gives the lung a tendency to elastic recoil which is important in the mechanism of breathing. This elasticity, or capacity of the lung to stretch, is known as compliance.

MEDIASTINUM

The mediastinum is the space between the two lungs and contains the heart and great vessels, trachea and oesophagus, phrenic and vagus nerves and lymph nodes.

PLEURA AND PLEURAL CAVITIES

The pleura is a continuous serous membrane that totally covers the surface of the lungs and the inner surface of the thoracic cavity. The visceral pleura lines the surface of the lungs, and the parietal pleura lines the thoracic wall and the upper surface of the diaphragm.

The tiny space between the parietal and visceral pleural layers is called the pleural cavity and contains a thin film of serous fluid. This fluid containing cavity has two functions. It lubricates the pleural surfaces so that as the lungs expand and contract during breathing, there is no friction. It also helps the two surfaces to bond so that the lungs are able to move with the chest wall during breathing. In reality there is actually no cavity and it is sometimes referred to as a potential space which enlarges in certain disease states. For example, it may contain blood (haemothorax), fluid (pleural effusion) or air (pneumothorax).

THE THORAX

The lower part of the trachea, the bronchi and the lungs are contained within the thorax together with the heart and major vessels, and the oesophagus. The thorax is a cone-shaped structure, the widest part being at the bottom where it sits on the diaphragm. It is protected by the ribcage.

THE MUSCLES OF RESPIRATION

We have mentioned the bronchial smooth muscle several times in describing the structure and function of the airways. There are other muscles, however, that are equally important in the process of respiration which are discussed below.

THE DIAPHRAGM

The diaphragm is the main muscle of respiration and sits at the base of the lungs. It is usually concave in shape; however, in conditions where air trapping occurs, for example chronic obstructive pulmonary disease (COPD) the diaphragm becomes flatter. This is sometimes obvious on chest X-ray. The right side of the diaphragm is slightly higher than the left to accommodate the liver situated underneath. Several important structures pass through the diaphragm:

- the inferior vena cava
- the oesophagus
- the aorta

THE INTERCOSTAL MUSCLES

The intercostal muscles span the space between each rib, and their main function is to hold the ribs together. However, in respiration they have another part to play which is discussed in the next section on the mechanics of breathing.

THE MECHANISM OF BREATHING

During quiet inspiration the diaphragm descends and becomes flatter, the intercostal muscles move the lower ribs outwards and upwards, and the sternum and upper ribs forwards and upwards. This results in expansion of the chest leading to air being drawn in by a negative intrathoracic pressure, that is air drawn from an area of high pressure to an area of low pressure. The air at the entrance to the respiratory system is atmospheric air, and the air in the lungs is alveolar air. We cannot change the pressure of atmospheric air, so the pressure of alveolar air governs this process. When alveolar air pressure falls, air is sucked in to the lungs to equalize the pressure.

During quiet expiration, the intercostal muscles relax, the diaphragm and ribs fall back to their original position and air is pushed out. This is a passive movement and the air is driven out mainly by the elastic recoil of the lungs. In normal health the respiratory rate for adults is 12–18 breaths per minute, and in children, 18–20 breaths per minute. The respiratory rate, however, can alter in response to activities such as vigorous exercise, or crying and laughing.

In adults, about eight litres of air are drawn into the lungs each minute, 25 % of which remains in the airways and so is not available for gas exchange. This is known as the anatomical dead space and comprises all the airways from the nose and mouth, right down to the terminal bronchioles. The volume is usually about 150 ml, but this can vary depending on the body size, and also can change with increased levels of inspiration. Another area where dead space may occur is in the alveoli. In certain disease states, for example emphysema, the alveoli are damaged and therefore unable to take part in gas exchange. This is known as the physiological dead space. In normal health, the anatomical and physiological dead space are equal, but where there is damage to the alveoli, the physiological dead space increases and the volume can be up to 10 times greater than that of anatomical dead space.

In forced inspiration and expiration, as sometimes happens in an acute asthma attack, other muscles come into play which fix the scapulae and the arms. If you have ever seen someone with extreme breathlessness, you may have noticed the position they adopt, with shoulders raised and fixed, and hands perhaps grasping the knees or the back of a chair. In addition other muscles force the contraction of the abdominal wall, thus pushing up the diaphragm. These are known as the accessory muscles of respiration.

CONTROL OF RESPIRATION

Going back to the introduction to this chapter, it was stated that the main function of the respiratory system is to maintain the balance of carbon dioxide and oxygen in the body. This is a very finely tuned process, and controlled by the respiratory centre, situated in the medulla oblongata in the brainstem. It is mainly an involuntary process, because obviously, you don't have to remember to breathe, it just happens. Messages pass from the respiratory centre in the brain to the nerves and muscles of the respiratory system, resulting in either an inspiration of air, or expiration, whichever is needed. The respiratory centre comes under the control of the nervous system which is divided into two subsystems: the autonomic nervous system, which is involuntary, and the somatic nervous system which is voluntary.

The bronchial smooth muscle in the airways, and the diaphragm and intercostal muscles, are controlled by the autonomic nervous system, because as previously stated, breathing is an involuntary act. However, it does not end there. The autonomic nervous system is further divided into the sympathetic and parasympathetic nervous systems, and the way these relate to breathing control is demonstrated in Figure 2.4.

The sympathetic nervous system comes into play when we find ourselves in a situation with which we are not happy, for example when confronted with a bull in a field. Do we run away, or do we stop and fight? I suspect the former is more likely. The message travels along the nerve pathway until it reaches the gap, or synapse, at the nerve ending. The chemical messenger adrenaline carries the message across to combine with receptors in the target tissue. In the lungs, the adrenaline combines with B2 receptors in the bronchial smooth muscle to open up the airways. The other actions of adrenaline include raising the blood pressure and increasing the heart rate. The increase in airway diameter, raised blood pressure and pulse rate enable us to run away, or fight as the case may be.

The parasympathetic nervous system helps to protect the airways against inhaled irritants such as smoke or dust. In this case the chemical messenger is acetylcholine which combines with cholinergic receptors in the bronchial smooth muscle to cause bronchoconstriction.

These two effects are demonstrated in Figures 2.5 and 2.6.

The actions of the sympathetic and parasympathetic nervous systems are very important because many drugs used in the management of asthma act on these systems. This is discussed in more detail in Chapter 5.

So far we have discussed the role of the nervous system in the way we breathe. There are other factors, however, which are also important in this process. In normal

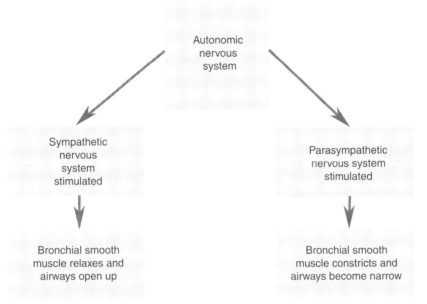

Figure 2.4. The autonomic nervous system and its effect on breathing control.

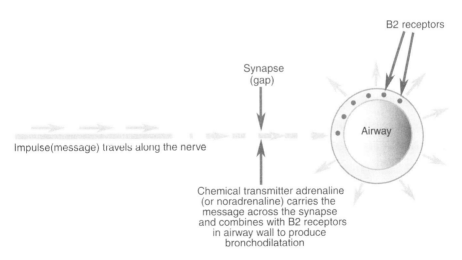

Figure 2.5. Effect of stimulation of the sympathetic nervous system.

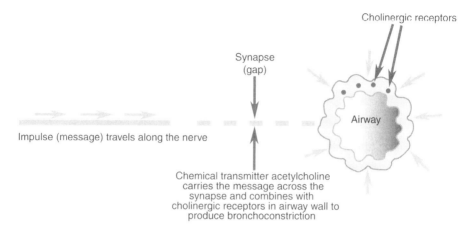

Figure 2.6. Effect of stimulation of the parasympathetic nervous system.

health, a change in the levels of carbon dioxide in the body is the most important factor in the control of ventilation. There are sensors located all over the body which detect even the minutest imbalance, and alert the respiratory centre in the brain that we either need to breathe in, or breathe out, to correct the disparity. The process by which this happens is known as pulmonary diffusion, when oxygen and carbon dioxide are exchanged in the lungs.

Control of breathing in this way is known as metabolic control – the respiratory system responds to metabolic changes in our bodies. However, there is also a behavioural control, when the metabolic control can be overridden. This happens in situations when we hold our breath, sing, cough or laugh, for example. We are also able to make ourselves breathe faster or more slowly. This is obviously a voluntary control.

Before going on to discuss pulmonary diffusion, we need to remind ourselves of the pulmonary circulation and the part it plays in the respiratory process. Blood, depleted of oxygen, enters the right side of the heart via the inferior and superior vena cava. From here it is transported by the pulmonary arteries to the pulmonary circulation where it picks up oxygen. The blood then travels through the pulmonary veins to re-enter the heart on the left side. This process is known as pulmonary perfusion. From the left side of the heart, oxygenated blood is taken by the aorta and carried around the body, thereby distributing oxygen to the tissues, to re-enter the right side of the heart and begin the whole process again. This is illustrated in Figure 2.7.

Occasionally, patients with severe respiratory disease develop right-sided heart failure, also known as cor pulmonale. This is caused by prolonged high blood pressure in the pulmonary artery and right ventricle of the heart. In normal health, the blood pressure is much higher on the left side of the heart than it is on the right side of the heart, in order to pump the blood around the body. When there is prolonged high blood pressure in the arteries and veins of the lungs, as happens in severe lung

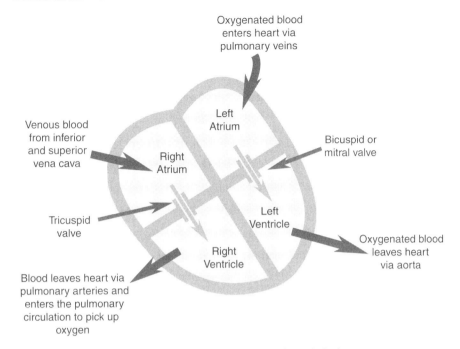

Figure 2.7. Illustration of blood flow through the heart.

disease, this causes back pressure on the right side of the heart leading to heart failure secondary to lung disease.

PULMONARY DIFFUSION

Gas exchange takes place in the alveoli which are the terminal points in the bronchial tree. They are surrounded by a dense network of capillaries. The blood in these capillaries picks up oxygen from the alveoli to be transported round the body, and transfers carbon dioxide back to the alveoli to be excreted. The capillary endothelium and alveolar epithelium are extremely thin and made up of a single layer of cells, which allows diffusion to take place. Diffusion is the process by which molecules pass from an area of greater concentration to an area of lower concentration. In gas exchange this means that oxygen moves from the alveoli to the capillaries where most of it binds with haemoglobin to form oxyhaemoglobin. The carbon dioxide from the cells combines with water in the blood, and after various chemical changes, finally breaks down again into water and carbon dioxide in the alveoli and is exhaled.

The small portion of oxygen which does not bind with haemoglobin dissolves in plasma, which can be measured as the partial pressure of oxygen in arterial blood. You may have seen this written on arterial blood gas analysis reports as PaO_2.

In normal states, central chemoreceptors in the medulla oblongata respond to high levels of carbon dioxide to stimulate ventilation. In some conditions, for example COPD, patients often have constantly high levels of carbon dioxide, therefore the brain can no longer use this as a stimulus to breathe. When this happens, the respiratory centre in the brain has to find another way to stimulate ventilation. It does this by detecting low levels of oxygen which then become the stimulus for ventilation to take place.

This is extremely important to remember when giving oxygen to a patient with COPD. If the patient's stimulus to breathe is a result of having low levels of oxygen, and they are given high percentage oxygen, the brain does not get the message that ventilation should take place and the patient will stop breathing!

SUMMARY

This chapter has described the anatomy and physiology of the respiratory system in as simple a way as possible. Although this may be thought of as perhaps the most tedious part of learning, it is important, and it makes it so much more interesting when treating patients, to be able to link signs and symptoms with what is happening inside the body.

FURTHER READING

1. Bourke, S.J., Brewis, R.A.L. (1998) *Lecture Notes on Respiratory Medicine*, 5th edn, Blackwell Science, London.
2. McGowan, P., Jeffries, A., Turley, A. (2003) *Respiratory System*, 2nd edn, Elsevier Science Ltd., Philadelphia.

3   Asthma the Disease

Key points:

- Asthma was first described over 2700 years ago.
- The causes of asthma are not known, although it is known to run in families and is associated with other atopic conditions such as hay fever.
- The male sex is a risk factor for developing asthma in infancy.
- Asthma is a variable disease of the airways characterized by inflammation and airways constriction.
- The inflammatory process in asthma is highly complex and involves many inflammatory cells and mediators.
- Contact with an allergen leads to an increase in immunoglobulin E (IgE) which triggers the inflammatory response, leading to the symptoms of asthma.
- Many triggers for asthma have been identified, but not all asthmatics will be susceptible to the same triggers.
- The airway narrowing that occurs in asthma is usually reversible.
- Ongoing, uncontrolled inflammation can lead to structural changes in the airways, leading to airway wall remodelling, which is usually not responsive to treatment.

THE HISTORY OF ASTHMA

Asthma has been described since the early ages and was first mentioned by Homer in *The Iliad*, around 2700 years ago, when he talked about a warrior who died after a battle with 'asthma and perspiration'. The word asthma translates from the Greek for 'panting', or 'gasping for breath'. The Ebers Papyrus which was discovered in Egypt in the 1870s and dates back to 1550 BC, described over 700 remedies for various conditions, one of which was asthma. The treatment in this case was to inhale a mixture of herbs heated on a brick.

The name asthma was first used as a medical term in the writings of Hippocrates (*c*. 460–360 BC) During the centuries that followed, asthma was variously described as 'fluid pouring into the lungs from the brain', an imbalance of 'humours', and 'epilepsy of the lungs'. In the early part of the seventeenth century, the association between inhaled substances and worsening of the condition was recognized and also that it got worse in situations of stress and emotional disturbances. Wheezing was first noted in the nineteenth century by a French physician called Laennec who had invented the first stethoscope. Triggers for asthma were also identified during the nineteenth century by an English physician called Henry Salter. By the beginning of the twentieth century, the role of inflammation was beginning to be recognized together with the connection to other allergic-type conditions such as hay fever and conjunctivitis.

Unfortunately, during the early twentieth century, it was also noted that people who had bad, or uncontrolled asthma, were often depressed or anxious. Although this was probably as a result of worrying when their next asthma attack would occur, it led to such people being labelled as neurotic, with asthma being considered more of a psychological, rather than a physical condition. Fortunately, this opinion has changed over the years, and asthma is now recognized as being a physical condition of the lungs. However, stress and emotions can affect asthma control and can also trigger an acute asthma attack.

WHAT CAUSES ASTHMA?

When discussing the causes and triggers of asthma, it is important to differentiate between the two terms. The former relates to how and why an individual develops asthma. The latter relates to the influences that make asthma worse. To be susceptible to asthma triggers, you have to have asthma in the first place. The triggers are well known, but the causes are much more difficult to define.

Strictly speaking, we do not know what causes asthma. The prevalence has increased over the last thirty to forty years and a lot of work is being done to try to find out the reasons for this. It has been argued that clinicians are more likely to make a diagnosis of asthma now than they were previously. For example, what was once called wheezy bronchitis, or chest infections in childhood may have been asthma under another name.

There is evidence that asthma runs in families and is associated with other atopic conditions such as hay fever. It is also known that the association with atopy is more strongly related to the mother rather than the father. Atopy is the tendency to produce large amounts of immunoglobulin E (IgE) in response to contact with common antigens. There may also be a family history of eczema. The male sex is a risk factor for developing asthma in infancy, although during adolescence it is' more common in girls. It is not clear why this happens, and one theory put forward argues that the airway diameter of boys is smaller than girls at birth, and also during infancy, leading to increased susceptibility to airway hyperreactivity.

However, apart from genetics, there are other factors that contribute to the increase in prevalence, and these are thought to be much more closely related to the environment in which we live. One example of this theory was demonstrated in the early 1970s when people living on the Pacific atoll of Tokelau were evacuated to New Zealand following a typhoon which devastated the island. The prevalence of asthma increased among those who had been moved but stayed the same in those who remained on the island [1]. Following this, a study investigating why asthma prevalence on Tokelau was so much lower than in New Zealand found that allergen levels were significantly lower in homes on the island than in comparative homes in New Zealand [2]. The authors concluded that this was the reason for the much lower prevalence of asthma on the island than in New Zealand.

Another theory put forward is that perhaps, in our modern homes we are too clean. One hundred years ago, tap water was untreated, we did not use strong cleaners and disinfectants in our kitchens and bathrooms, and we did not have vaccination against common diseases. As a result, our parents and grandparents came into contact with a large variety of bacteria and diseases to which today's children are not exposed. This so-called 'hygiene hypothesis' argues that the body overreacts to contact with house dust mites and other allergens because it does not have the need to fight bacteria. Again this is a theory which has yet to be proven and much more research is needed to be able to state categorically the reasons for the increase in asthma.

Maternal smoking in pregnancy has been shown to lead to an increased risk of having a wheezy baby [3], and it has also been shown to have an adverse effect on lung function in early life [4]. The latter study also found that children who live in a smoking household are more at risk from having repeated chest infections and wheezing illnesses [4].

ASTHMA TRIGGERS

Many triggers have been identified for asthma, but not all asthmatics will be susceptible to the same triggers. The most common trigger in childhood is the common cold and many parents will say that their child only gets asthma symptoms when they get a cold. Contact with allergens such as house dust mite, pets and pollens will trigger asthma symptoms in susceptible people. Some people find that contact with allergens causes constant hay fever-like symptoms, for example itchy or runny eyes and nose. This is known as perennial rhinitis, and in contrast to normal hay fever, the symptoms of perennial rhinitis are present all year round and can be a big problem for some asthmatics. Issues surrounding allergen avoidance and house dust mite control are dealt with in detail in Chapter 7.

Quite often people with asthma find their symptoms get worse during, or after, vigorous exercise, and if this happens, using a short-acting B2 agonist 15–30 min before exercise will often help.

There are three groups of drugs that may trigger asthma in susceptible people. These are aspirin, nonsteroidal anti-inflammatory drugs (NSAIDs) and beta blockers. Beta blockers are often given for hypertension, but also used in eye drops for the treatment of glaucoma. B2 receptors are found in bronchial smooth muscle, and when these are stimulated the muscle relaxes, thereby opening up the airways. Blocking the action of B2 receptors therefore can provoke asthma symptoms in some people. A small percentage of asthmatics will be sensitive to aspirin and NSAIDs. Even topical preparations such as the gels used to treat soft tissue inflammation can trigger an asthma attack in susceptible people.

Table 3.1. Common asthma triggers

Common asthma triggers	
Viral infections, for example colds	Pregnancy and menstruation
Pets/animals	Some drugs
Pollen	House dust mite
Stress/emotion	Food allergies
Smoking	Cold air
Fumes	Hot air
Spores	
Exercise	

Occasionally, asthma may be triggered by foods, the most common of which are dairy products, shellfish and nuts. However, food allergy triggering asthma is relatively rare and it is important that parents of young children do not start removing foods from the diet without speaking to their doctor or nurse first. If it is confirmed that a child does have a food allergy, they should be referred to a dietician for expert advice.

Stress and emotion are also known to trigger the symptoms of asthma in some people. Great sensitivity is needed in dealing with this type of asthma, because in the past it was often thought that asthma was a psychological condition. Even today, many people believe asthma is a hysterical response to being unable to cope with difficult situations. There is no doubt that psychological influences do have a part to play in asthma, and this will be discussed in more detail in Chapter 8. However, irrespective of the triggers, the symptoms of asthma are very real and should always be treated as such. Remember also that children with asthma are often triggered by exciting events such as birthday parties, or Christmas.

Some women find that their asthma symptoms are related to their menstrual cycle, and pregnancy can also be a problem for some women. These issues are discussed in more depth in Chapter 8.

Table 3.1 lists the most common triggers in asthma, but it should be remembered that this list is not exhaustive and that anything can trigger asthma in susceptible individuals.

WHAT IS ASTHMA?

Asthma is a disease of the airways characterized by inflammation and airway constriction. The main feature of asthma that differentiates it from other lung diseases such as COPD is its variability. The British Thoracic Society [5] uses the following definition which has been taken from the International Consensus Report of 1992: [6] Asthma is:

a chronic inflammatory disorder of the airways ... in susceptible individuals, inflammatory symptoms are usually associated with widespread but variable airflow obstruction and an increase in airway response to a variety of stimuli. Obstruction is often reversible, either spontaneously or with treatment.

The pathogenesis of asthma is very complex involving a number of factors. Basically, inflammation in the airways causes bronchial hyperreactivity which leads to a whole chain of events culminating in the symptoms of asthma. This event is usually triggered by exposure to an allergen such as pollen or house dust mite.

THE ROLE OF INFLAMMATION

In susceptible individuals, the inhalation of an allergen leads to a highly complex chain of events which eventually results in the symptoms of asthma. In the past, it was thought that the inflammation that occurred in asthma was only present during acute episodes. It has now become clear that inflammation is constantly present to a greater or lesser degree in all patients with asthma, and that it is related to the levels of airway hyperresponsiveness that the patient might experience.

When an asthmatic patient inhales an allergen, for example pollens or fumes, the body's immune response goes into overdrive and causes the production of large quantities of immunoglobulin E (IgE). IgE is an important aspect of the inflammatory process and leads to the airway walls becoming infiltrated with inflammatory cells, such as mast cells, macrophages and eosinophils. Other inflammatory cells include T-lymphocytes, epithelial cells and neutrophils. Mast cells initiate the bronchoconstricting response and are also thought to play a part in the airway narrowing that occurs with exercise-induced asthma. Eosinophils are key components of the inflammatory process in asthma, and following activation in the airways they release mediators such as leukotrienes, histamine and prostaglandins. These mediators constrict the bronchial smooth muscle, increase airway mucus secretion and attract other inflammatory cells.

This process is illustrated in Figure 3.1.

These aforementioned mediators are important aspects of the inflammation that occurs in acute asthma; however, other mediators, called cytokines, are thought to be more important in the chronic inflammation that is often present in asthmatic patients. Cytokines consist of a number of interleukins which are numbered IL-1 to IL-33, each one having a different function. Some of the more important interleukins in asthma include IL-4, which is involved with the development of T-cells and mast cells, and IL-9, which stimulates mast cell production. Cytokines can be produced by every cell in certain conditions and, in chronic asthma, help to promote the inflammatory process even further.

As stated previously, the whole process of inflammation is very complex and no single inflammatory cell or mediator can be held responsible for the chain of events that occurs. It is more likely that a combination of factors leads to the development of inflammation which may vary from person to person, depending on which cells and mediators have been activated. Inflammation, however, is only one aspect of the symptoms of asthma, and the inflammatory response that follows exposure to an allergen leads on to another chain of events, resulting in airway narrowing. This effect is known as bronchial hyperreactivity. It can be split into two types, the early response and the late response. In reality most asthmatics will show evidence of both, although one or the other of them may be absent.

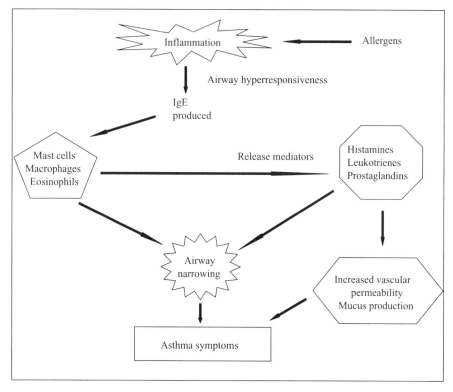

Figure 3.1. The effect of an allergen on the inflammatory process in asthma.

BRONCHIAL HYPERREACTIVITY

Bronchial hyperreactivity, also sometimes called bronchial hyperresponsiveness, is the response of the airways to inhaled irritants. For example, most people will cough when coming into contact with dust or smoke. This is a protective reflex and is the result of stimulation of the parasympathetic nervous system, when the chemical messenger acetylcholine combines with cholinergic receptors in the bronchial smooth muscle to produce bronchoconstriction. Bronchial smooth muscle is present in all the airways, and constriction of this muscle results in narrowing of the airway leading to the symptoms of breathlessness, cough and wheeze. In addition to this, extra mucus is produced by the goblet cells in the airway walls to enable the irritants to be transported upwards by the cilia to the pharynx where they will be either coughed up or swallowed.

In nonasthmatics the episode is usually quickly dealt with. The person leaves the environment and the airways rapidly return to normal without any need for treatment. However, in asthma, the way the airways react to the same irritant is highly exaggerated, and it will take longer for someone with asthma to recover and they may need treatment.

EARLY RESPONSE

Exposure to an allergen causes large quantities of the antibody immunoglobulin E (IgE) to be produced. The IgE combines and interacts with receptors on inflammatory cells, most notably the mast cells found in the bronchial epithelium. This interaction causes the release of preformed mediators such as histamine and prostaglandins. Neutral proteases and chemotactic factors for neutrophils and eosinophils are also released. The term chemotaxis refers to the movement of cells induced by a chemotactic stimulus. Other substances released include tissue necrosis factor and a set of lipid mediators, including leukotrienes.

This process is called mast cell degranulation, and causes vascular permeability leading to bronchial oedema and smooth muscle constriction. If you remember from the section on anatomy and physiology, the lining of the airways contains a layer of smooth muscle, so when this muscle constricts as a result of mast cell degranulation, the airways become narrow.

This early reaction occurs within minutes of contact with the allergen, peaks at about 10–15 min and lasts about 1–2 h. It is much easier to reverse than the later reaction, which usually occurs about 6–12 h following exposure to the allergen.

LATE RESPONSE

The late response usually happens about 6–12 h following the initial exposure to the trigger; however, it can occur up to 24 h later. A whole new chain of events now takes place. Bronchial oedema becomes more marked and the mast cells in the bronchial epithelium release cytokines and chemokines to the mucosal layer. These in turn attract eosinophils, basophils and macrophages which promote further inflammation, thus amplifying the allergic response.

This process can often be identified in a patient's peak flow rate which usually falls dramatically at initial exposure to an allergen, and then improves with treatment. Several hours later, the peak flow rate will fall again at the start of the late response. This is illustrated in Figure 3.2. Note the sudden drop in peak flow and gradual increase of the early response and then the repeated drop of peak flow in the late response.

The airway narrowing in the late response is often much more difficult to reverse than the airway narrowing in the early response, and can persist for several weeks.

AIRWAY WALL REMODELLING

Repeated acute episodes of asthma, or ongoing inflammation, that is not controlled can result in structural changes to the airways. As a result of oedema, and cellular infiltration, the basement membrane becomes significantly thicker. The bronchial smooth muscle and mucous glands hypertrophy leading to fibrosis of the airway wall, resulting in increased bronchial sensitivity and permanent narrowing of the airways. These structural changes to the airway are not responsive to bronchodilator

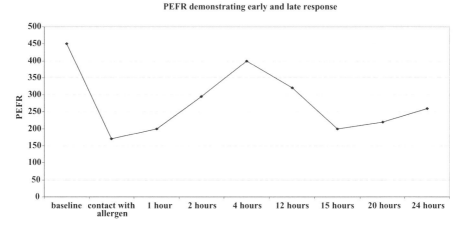

Figure 3.2. Chart illustrating peak flow in the early and late asthmatic response.

therapy and lead to gradual deterioration in lung function. The process is known as airway wall remodelling, and can be exacerbated by other factors such as smoking. As time goes on the asthma will change from being a reversible condition to become chronic obstructive pulmonary disease which is a fixed airways condition.

SUMMARY

Asthma has been in existence for at least 2700 years, although it was not until the nineteenth century that we really started to gain any understanding about its development and effects. We now have a much greater understanding of the pathology of asthma, but unfortunately the causes of asthma are still largely a mystery.

The role of inflammation, and its effect on the airways, has been discussed at length because it is the single most important aspect of asthma. The inflammatory process is very complex, but when you have an understanding of the way it behaves in the patient with asthma, and the effect it has on the lungs and airways, the easier, and more interesting, it will be to manage your patients effectively.

REFERENCES

1. Crane, J., O'Donnell, T.V., Prior, I.A., Waite, D.A. (1989) The relationship between atopy, bronchial hyperresponsiveness, and a family history of asthma: a cross-sectional study of migrant Tokelauan children in New Zealand. *Journal of Allergy and Clinical Immunology*, **84** (5 Pt 1), 768–72.
2. Lane, J., Siebers, R., Pene, G., *et al.* (2005) Tokelau: a unique low allergen environment at sea level. *Clinical and Experimental Allergy*, **35** (4), 479–82.

3. Dezateau, C., Stocks, J., Dundas, I., Fletcher, M.E. (1999) Impaired airway function and wheezing in infancy: the influence of maternal smoking and a genetic predisposition to asthma. *American Journal of Respiratory and Critical Care Medicine*, **159** (2), 403–10.
4. Stocks, J., Dezateau, C. (2003) The effect of parental smoking on lung function and development during infancy. *Respirology*, **8** (3), 266–85.
5. British Thoracic Society/Scottish Intercollegiate Guidelines Network (2005) *British Guideline on the Management of Asthma*, Revised edition. Available at www.brit-thoracic.org.uk/guidelines.html.
6. International consensus report on diagnosis and treatment of asthma (1992) National Heart, Lung and Blood Institute, National Institutes of Health. Bethesda, Maryland 20892. Publication no. 92-3091, March 1992. *European Respiratory Journal*, **5** (5), 601–41.

FURTHER READING

7. Marketos, S.G., Ballas, C.N. (1982) Bronchial asthma in the medical literature of Greek antiquity. *Journal of Asthma*, **19** (4), 263–9.
8. Hopkin, J. (2003) Mechanisms of asthma. *Medicine*, **31**, 41–4.

4 The Presentation and Diagnosis of Asthma

Key points:

- The clinical features of asthma are cough, wheeze, breathlessness, tight chest and mucus production.
- Symptoms of asthma are typically worse at night and following exercise.
- In children, a night-time cough may be the only symptom.
- A diagnosis of asthma is based on a good clinical history and confirmed by objective measurements of peak flow or spirometry.
- It is important to always consider the possibility of alternative diagnoses.

INTRODUCTION

To be able to manage asthma effectively, you have to get the diagnosis right. This may sound obvious, but so often, patients either go undiagnosed or a wrong diagnosis is made. This can have disastrous effects on the patient, not to mention the difficulties it will cause you if you get it wrong. This chapter guides you through the signs and symptoms that suggest asthma and the process that ultimately leads to a diagnosis. Alternative diagnoses are also discussed.

THE CLINICAL FEATURES OF ASTHMA

The main symptoms of asthma are:

- cough
- wheeze
- tight chest
- breathlessness
- mucus production

Typically these symptoms are worse at night and following exercise. However, not everyone with asthma will have all these symptoms, especially children, when a night-time cough may be the only presenting feature. The important thing to remember when making a diagnosis is that asthma is a variable condition, which means it can change from day to day, or even from night to day. This differentiates it from a fixed airways disease such as chronic obstructive pulmonary disease (COPD), so it is important to ask both the right questions and to interpret tests correctly. Unless you have a high index of suspicion, there is always the risk that the diagnosis of asthma will be missed, which may in turn lead to unnecessary suffering for the patient and long-term lung problems which will be more difficult to treat.

COUGH

Cough is probably the most common presenting symptom of asthma. In children, it is often the only presenting symptom. The cough may be dry, or it may be productive. Typically people with asthma tend to cough more at night or with exercise, so it is important to find out when the cough is worse, or if there are any known precipitating factors, such as contact with allergens.

WHEEZE

Often people with asthma will not wheeze unless they come into contact with a trigger, or have an acute asthma attack. It is caused by air trying to get through narrowed air passages that are clogged up by mucus. Occasionally, during a severe asthma attack, the wheeze will disappear altogether because there is insufficient air moving in and out of the airways. This is a very serious sign in acute asthma and may lead to respiratory arrest.

TIGHT CHEST

Asking a patient to describe a tight chest can be quite difficult. Some say it is a feeling like someone sitting on their chest, or having a band tied around their chest. For others it may be less perceptible, but it leaves them feeling uncomfortable and not quite knowing why. Don't forget that young children can also experience this symptom, but are unable to communicate how they are feeling. Sometimes they say they have a tummy ache or even a sore throat. They may feel irritable leading to disruptive behaviour, which is often misconstrued as being naughty. This issue is discussed in more detail in Chapter 8.

BREATHLESSNESS

Patients with respiratory disease will often say that breathlessness is the most distressing symptom. Severe breathlessness is extremely frightening. It is important to determine the pattern of breathlessness to make sure of the right diagnosis. Breathlessness that occurs at night or in response to contact with an allergen is more indicative of asthma, whereas breathlessness that only occurs as a result of strenuous activity is more likely to be COPD.

The experience of breathlessness is very subjective and difficult to define. If you think about it, you are not always conscious of your breathing except when you are breathless, so one way of describing breathlessness may be to think of it as an increased awareness of the effort of breathing.

MUCUS PRODUCTION

Mucus production is a natural function of the mucociliary system, and normally about 100 ml is produced every day. In certain disease states this can increase to as much as 1 litre a day. People with asthma rarely produce excessive mucus except when they have an acute attack. During an attack, the mucus secreting glands in the airways multiply causing an increase in the amount of mucus produced. Occasionally asthmatic patients may cough up plugs of mucus cast in the shape of a smaller airway.

The mucus in asthma is usually clear, but can become discoloured during an exacerbation because of the increase in the number of eosinophils. This can be confusing, and may lead the clinician to think that there is infection present. The colour of the mucus during an exacerbation is not a reliable indication of infection, and very often patients are given unnecessary antibiotics for an acute episode of asthma, when what is needed is a course of steroid tablets.

Don't forget that these symptoms may not all be apparent, and also that they may appear or disappear at different times of the day or night, or even at different times of the year.

ASSESSMENT AND DIAGNOSIS

The clinical diagnosis of asthma is based on an accurate history and is usually confirmed with objective measurements of either peak flow or spirometry. However, in young children, objective measurements are not always possible except in specialist centres, so careful history-taking is even more important. Physical examination at the time of diagnosis may not be helpful as airway obstruction may not be present at that time.

TAKING A HISTORY

When taking a clinical history in order to make a diagnosis, it is best to follow a standard procedure or protocol so that you do not forget anything. A good history will include the following:

Symptoms

- What are the symptoms?
- When did they start?

- When do they most often occur?
- Was it a sudden onset or a more gradual onset?
- Does anything make them worse?
- Does anything make them better?
- What are the current symptoms?

It is also important to ask about smoking history, past and present. When asked, very often patients will say they do not smoke, but will omit to tell you about the 50 cigarettes a day they smoked when they were in their twenties. This will have a bearing on your final diagnosis, when trying to differentiate between asthma and COPD.

Family History

- Do any close family members have asthma, hay fever or eczema?
- Do any close family members have any form of respiratory disease?
- Does anyone in the household smoke?

Allergies

- Are there any known allergies?
- Are there allergies to any drugs?

Additional useful information will include things like current medications, including over the counter drugs, just in case any of these may be contributing to their symptoms. The triggers for asthma are discussed more fully in Chapter 3. It is also important to find out whether the patient's occupation is a possible cause for their symptoms. The section on occupational asthma in Chapter 8 deals with this subject in detail. In children it is also important to check height and weight, and compare these to predicted values for their age.

PHYSICAL EXAMINATION

Nurses are generally becoming more skilled in examining patients, and you may feel you have the necessary skills and knowledge to perform a chest examination. However, a physical examination in the diagnosis of asthma is not always necessary and will not be helpful unless the patient is exhibiting signs or symptoms of respiratory distress at the time. There are some signs and symptoms that are obvious without doing any form of examination. You do not need a stethoscope to hear a cough, for example, and sometimes a wheeze can be audible to the 'naked' ear.

Look out for other clues to aid you in your diagnosis. Observe how the patient is behaving. Do they appear anxious or relaxed? Are they breathless or wheezy? Check skin colour, look for hyperexpansion of the thorax, use of accessory muscles and any chest wall deformity.

DIAGNOSTIC TESTS AND THEIR MEANINGS

Let us suppose that you have taken a full history and feel fairly sure that the patient has asthma. The next step is to try to prove this with some objective tests. We have already discussed the fact that asthma is a variable condition, which means that the airways of an asthmatic person will become narrow, or widen, in response to certain stimuli. We can now use this characteristic to aid us in the diagnostic process.

OBJECTIVE MEASUREMENTS OF LUNG FUNCTION

The first thing you will need to do is to get some reliable lung function results. There are two available methods for measuring lung function and the choice will depend on the availability of equipment and expertise of the practitioner. It should be remembered however, that a single reading can be misleading due to the variability of the condition as previously discussed.

PEAK EXPIRATORY FLOW RATE (PEFR)

The most common and easiest way of measuring lung function is to use a peak flow meter. It is relatively easy to use, both for the nurse and the patient, and is cheap and convenient. It also has the advantage of being available on prescription, so the patient can monitor their own peak flows at home. A peak flow meter measures the rate at which the patient can forcibly exhale air, in litres per minute, so it follows that the narrower the airway, the lower the reading will be. However, there are also disadvantages with using a peak flow meter. It only measures how fast air can be blown out through the larger airways, so it does not give much information about lung capacities and what is happening in the lower airways. The results are also not as reproducible as a spirometry test. A typical peak flow meter is illustrated in Figure 4.1.

Most children under the age of five years are unable to do a reliable peak flow, so in this age group diagnosis and management is centred around symptom control, rather than on objective measurements. It is also important not to confuse a child by asking them to blow into one device, a peak flow meter, and then suck in with another device, an inhaler. If they need inhaled therapy, it is much more important that they are able to use their inhaler than blow into a peak flow meter.

Method for Taking a Peak Flow Measurement

- Stand up if possible.
- Ensure the cursor is on zero.
- Take a deep breath in.
- Put the mouthpiece in the mouth and make a good seal with the lips around the mouthpiece.

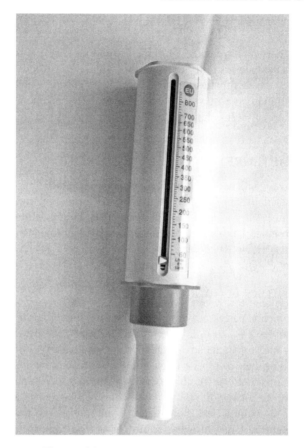

Figure 4.1. Photograph of a peak flow meter.

- Blow as hard and fast as possible.
- Check the number indicated by the cursor.
- Return the cursor to zero.
- Repeat twice more and record the highest reading.

Before you do a peak flow measurement you will need to know the patient's age, height and sex. The reading can then be compared to the predicted value for someone with the same characteristics. A single peak flow reading, however, will not tell you if the patient has asthma or not. Remember, asthma is a variable condition, so the peak flow may well be normal at 2 o'clock in the afternoon, but this gives no indication as to what it was at 2 o'clock in the morning. Charts of predicted values are commonly available and easy to read. In children, you will only need to know the child's height. It is important to remember, however, that many patients' normal peak flow will not conform with predicted values. For example, someone with a predicted peak flow rate

---

Gary's story

Gary is twenty-five years old and has had asthma since early childhood. Most of the time it is well controlled on an inhaled steroid and long-acting bronchodilator, both of which he takes twice daily. Occasionally he needs to take a short-acting bronchodilator for exercise-induced symptoms. Gary is a keen sportsman, and plays football for his local team. Gary's predicted peak flow rate, calculated from his age, height and sex is 660 litres per minute. However, Gary regularly records measurements much higher than this, his best peak flow being 740 litres per minute.

One Saturday, following a football match, Gary is brought into A & E by some of his team mates because they were worried about his breathing, and he was coughing and wheezing. On assessment he was found to have a peak flow rate of 500 l/min which is 75% of his predicted value. On the basis of this assessment he was treated as per BTS Guidelines as having a mild exacerbation. He was given a nebulized bronchodilator and discharged from the department. What had not been recognized, however, was the fact that Gary's normal best peak flow is 740 l/min, which would mean his peak flow on admission to the department was actually only 67% of his best result. This would put Gary into the moderate category and should have alerted the A & E staff that Gary was more at risk than they had previously thought.

As a result of this misunderstanding, Gary was brought in again to the A & E Department later on that evening with a severe asthma attack, and had to be admitted to hospital. If this episode had been treated more vigorously in the first place, the chances are that Gary would not have ended up in hospital.

Figure 4.2. Gary's story.

of 540 l/min may regularly blow 600 l/min. This could be misleading as illustrated in Figure 4.2.

SPIROMETRY

Although more difficult to perform, spirometry does give much more reliable and meaningful results. Put simply, it measures the amount of air that can be forcibly exhaled from the lungs in one second, that is, the forced expiratory volume in one second (FEV1), and the total amount of air that can be forcibly exhaled, that is, the forced vital capacity (FVC). By comparing these results with the patient's predicted measurements, it is possible to reliably diagnose airway obstruction. There are many different types of spirometer available and Figure 4.3 shows a typical portable spirometer that is commonly used in general practice. There are much larger versions available which are generally used in hospitals.

Method for Doing a Spirometry Test

Before you start doing a spirometry test, there are certain criteria that need to be followed to ensure you have a safe, reliable test. This criteria is taken from the *Guidelines for the Measurement of Respiratory Function*, published by the

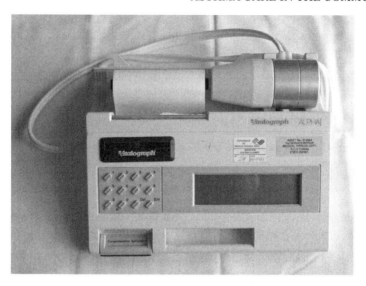

Figure 4.3. Photograph of a portable spirometer.

British Thoracic Society and the Association of Respiratory Technicians and Physiologists [1].

- The patient should be clinically stable.
- The patient should not have taken a short-acting B2 agonist within the preceding four hours, or an anticholinergic within the preceding six hours, or a long-acting B2 agonist within the preceding twelve hours.
- The patient should not be wearing any restrictive clothing such as a corset.
- The patient should remove any loose-fitting dentures.
- The patient should be seated, preferably in a chair with arms, in case of any faintness or dizziness while doing the test.

You will need to make a note of the patient's age, height, sex and ethnic origin, in order to compare the results to the predicted values for someone with the same characteristics. If you have an electronic machine which does all the calculations for you, this information must be entered into the machine before you start the test. You are then ready to perform the test.

- Explain the test to the patient (you may need to demonstrate the technique).
- Ask the patient to take a deep breath in and put the mouthpiece in the mouth, making sure there is a good seal with the lips around the mouthpiece.
- Ask the patient to blow out as hard and fast as possible, and also to keep blowing out as long as possible.
- Repeat the above, giving the patient time to recover between each blow. A maximum of eight attempts can be made in one session.

To ensure accuracy and reliability of the test, at least three technically accurate readings should be obtained and two FEV1 readings should be within 5 % of each other. Spirometry is a very important test of lung function, so it is vital that it is done properly. Patients quite often find it difficult to do, particularly when they have severe lung disease. Some common faults include coughing while blowing out, taking an extra breath or hesitation at the start of the test. If the test is less than perfect it should be stopped and the patient given a chance to recover before trying again. In clinical practice, however, you may well find that no matter how much instruction you give the patient, or how well you demonstrate the technique, some people are just not able to perform an accurate and reliable test.

Interpreting Spirometry Results

Once you have got a reliable spirometry test, you need to be able to understand what it is telling you. The first thing to look at is the graph, which shows lung volume over time. In normal health it is usually possible to be able to expel all the air out of the lungs in the first four or five seconds. People with severe obstructive lung disease, however, as in COPD, take much longer, and can keep going for up to twenty seconds. So, the time taken to breathe out all the air in the lungs, and the shape of the curve will give you a lot of information before you start working out measurements. Figure 4.4 shows a normal lung tracing, an obstructive lung tracing and a restrictive lung tracing.

Look at the normal lung tracing first and note the steep climb of the curve as the patient starts to blow out as hard and as fast as they possibly can. The curve gently tapers off until there is no air left in the lungs and the patient stops blowing. The obstructive lung function graph shows a patient trying to blow out as hard as possible, but because the airways are narrow, they are not able to get very much air out in the first second, so the curve climbs much more gently. The eventual amount blown out is often normal as demonstrated in this graph, but it takes the patient very much longer to get to that point. The restrictive lung function graph looks very similar to

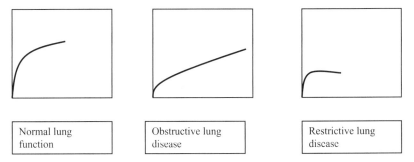

| Normal lung function | Obstructive lung disease | Restrictive lung disease |

Figure 4.4. Volume/time graphs showing the difference between normal lung function, obstructive lung disease and restrictive lung disease.

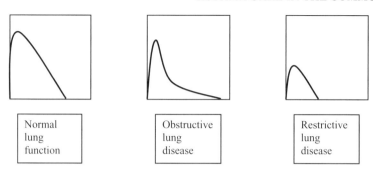

Figure 4.5. Flow/volume graphs showing the difference between normal lung function, obstructive lung disease and restrictive lung disease.

the normal graph, but a lot smaller. This is because in restrictive lung disease, there is usually a much smaller volume of air in the lungs to start off with, so the patient is able to blow it all out very quickly.

Asthma is an obstructive condition, as is COPD. Restrictive conditions include pulmonary fibrosis, fibrosing alveolitis and lung tumours. They are mentioned briefly at the end of this chapter under alternative diagnoses, but it is beyond the scope of this book to explore these conditions fully. Suffice it to say that if a spirometry result shows a restrictive pattern, the patient should be referred for further investigation and clarification of diagnosis.

Some spirometers will also produce another graph, called the flow volume curve. This measures airflow against volume, and again the shape of this graph will tell you a great deal about lung function without looking at the measurements. Figure 4.5 shows a normal lung volume curve, an obstructive lung volume curve and a restrictive lung volume curve.

A normal flow volume curve is roughly the shape of a triangle. Note the dip in the curve of the obstructive pattern. This happens because as the patient starts to blow out hard and fast, the airways collapse, leading to the characteristic 'church steeple effect' in obstructive airways disease. As in the volume/time graph, the restrictive flow volume curve is very similar in shape to the normal curve, but is much smaller. This can be quite confusing if you are not experienced in reading spirometry results, so it is important to view the results in conjunction with the clinical history before making a decision about treatment.

The next things you will need to look at are the actual measurements produced from the spirometry test, and compare them to their predicted values. As with peak flow measurements, predicted values are available, based on age, height and sex. In addition to this you will need to know the patient's ethnicity, as people from different races, black Africans or Asians for example, will have different predicted values. You may be lucky enough to have a spirometer that does all this for you, as in the one shown in Figure 4.3. Some surgeries, or clinics, however, may have the older version which only gives you a graph and you have to work everything out yourself.

Table 4.1. Lung function values

	Normal	Obstruction	Restriction
FVC	Above 80 % predicted	Above 80 % predicted	Below 80 % predicted
FEV1	Above 80 % predicted	Below 80 % predicted	Below 80 % predicted
FEV1/FVC %	Above 70 %	Below 70 %	Above 70 %

The results that a spirometry test will give you are shown below. Apart from the slow vital capacity (SVC) which is a separate measurement, the other three measurements are obtained from a single blow. SVC is not always recorded, as it is not considered to be as important as the other results. This is probably true in asthma, but when treating COPD, SVC is a very useful measurement.

- SVC = Slow vital capacity – the total amount of air that can be blown out in a slow, nonforced manner.
- FVC = Forced vital capacity – the total amount of air that can forcefully be blown out.
- FEV1 = Forced expiratory volume in one second – the amount of air that can forcefully be blown out in one second.
- FEV1/FVC% = the ratio of FEV1 to FVC expressed as a percentage.

The SVC, FVC and FEV1 are absolute values and measured in litres. In normal lung function, around 80 % of the total volume of air exhaled (FVC), can be blown out in the first second (FEV1). The narrower the airways, the lower this figure will be, and in very severe disease it can be as low as 15 %. Very often, the FVC will be normal, even in severe obstruction, but the patient will take longer to reach that point.

The ratio is calculated by dividing the patient's FEV1 by the FVC and multiplying by 100. When the airways are narrow, the FEV1 will be lower and therefore the ratio will be lower. A ratio of less than 70 % indicates obstruction. If the ratio is higher than 70 %, there is a possibility that the patient may have a restrictive disease, and should be referred for a definitive diagnosis.

Table 4.1 summarizes spirometry values for patients with normal, obstructive and restricted conditions.

> Remember: lung function results on their own are simply an aid to diagnosis and should only be used to confirm clinical findings.

Care and Maintenance of a Spirometer

To ensure accuracy and reliability, a spirometer needs to be looked after and serviced according to the manufacturer's recommendations. It should be kept clean and dust free, preferably in a relatively stable temperature. Some spirometers need to be calibrated using a large volume syringe, and again the manufacturer's recommendations should be followed as to how often this should be done.

REVERSIBILITY TEST

For both peak flow and spirometry tests there are standard predicted values for patients, which are calculated on their age, height and sex. In addition, when doing spirometry tests, you will also need to know the patient's ethnicity. If, when you do the test, you find that the results are below their predicted values, then the next step would be to do a reversibility test. The aim of this test is to find out if the patient responds to a bronchodilator, for example salbutamol.

Method for Performing a Reversibility Test

- Ensure the patient has had no short-acting bronchodilator in the preceding four hours, or long-acting bronchodilator in the preceding twelve hours.
- Measure baseline lung function results using a peak flow meter or spirometer.
- Administer a short-acting bronchodilator either by spacer device or nebulizer.
- Wait twenty minutes.
- Repeat lung function measurement.

To confirm a diagnosis of asthma there should be an improvement in the patient's lung function results. If using a peak flow meter, this improvement should be more than 20 % *and* 60 l/min, or, if using spirometry the FEV1 should improve by 15 % *and* at least 200 ml [2].

PEAK FLOW MONITORING

If a reversibility test is not possible or is inconclusive, the next step would be to do some home peak flow monitoring. The patient is given a peak flow meter and diary and asked to record their peak flow twice daily for two weeks. A variability of 20 % or more and a minimum change of at least 60 ml, ideally for three days in a week, is highly suggestive of asthma [2]. Figure 4.6 shows a diary of a typical peak flow pattern in someone with undiagnosed, or uncontrolled asthma.

REVERSIBILITY TO STEROID TABLETS

Another option in trying to decide 'is this asthma?' might be to do a steroid reversibility test. After obtaining the baseline measurements either by peak flow or spirometry, the patient is given 30 mg prednisolone daily for two weeks. Again the diagnosis is confirmed if there is an increase in peak flow of 20 % plus 60 l/min or an increase in FEV1 of 15 % plus 200 ml [2].

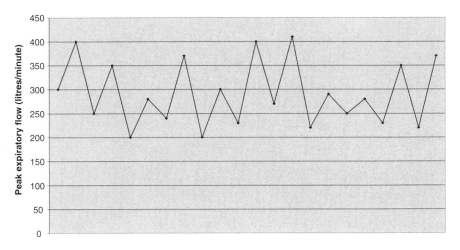

Figure 4.6. Typical pattern of peak flow in uncontrolled or undiagnosed asthma.

EXERCISE TEST

Another way of measuring airflow variability is to do an exercise test. In this test, after obtaining baseline measurements, the patient is asked to do six minutes of exercise, for example running or brisk walking. Lung function is then recorded every ten minutes for 30 min. As you are going to ask the patient to do five lung function tests, in addition to six minutes of exercise, it is probably better to use a peak flow meter in this instance. During exercise, the body produces large amounts of adrenaline, which if you remember causes an increase in pulse and blood pressure, and also relaxes bronchial smooth muscle resulting in the airways opening up. This will happen both in people who have asthma and in those who do not have asthma. However, the nonasthmatic's airways will quickly recover, whereas the asthmatic's airways will overreact and constrict following initial bronchodilatation. Figures 4.7a and b show what typically happens to peak flow in someone with exercise-induced asthma, and someone who does not have asthma.

> Be aware that an exercise test can sometimes produce asthma symptoms or even provoke a serious asthma attack. For this reason, exercise tests are not carried out so often in general practice. If you do decide that an exercise test is necessary, make sure that facilities for immediate treatment are at hand.

To demonstrate a typical diagnostic process, the following two scenarios illustrate the difference between asthma and another common lung disease, COPD. Although the symptoms in both are similar, note the differences in when they occur, Amy's symptoms (Figure 4.8) more often at night, and Bill's symptoms (Figure 4.9) more often during the day.

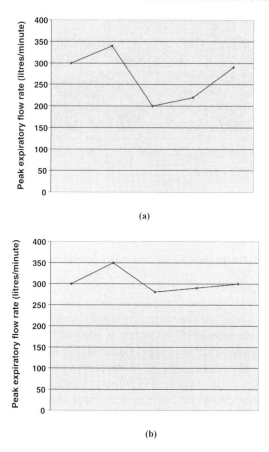

(a)

(b)

Figure 4.7. Typical pattern of peak flow in a patient with exercise-induced asthma (*a*) and in a nonasthmatic individual (*b*).

The diagnosis of asthma is usually straightforward as long as you use a consistent approach to the process. The procedures to follow are summarized in Figure 4.10 which shows a flow chart for the diagnosis of asthma.

DIAGNOSIS OF ASTHMA IN CHILDREN UNDER FIVE

It can be difficult to obtain a definitive diagnosis of asthma in young children as objective measurements of peak flow or spirometry are not possible. Asthma should be suspected in any child who presents with a wheezing-type illness, when

---

Amy's story

Amy is 10 years old and lives with her parents and younger brother. She goes to the local primary school and enjoys sports, especially swimming and tennis. Mum brings her to the surgery and says that over the last three to four months Amy has been coughing a lot, and seems tired and irritable. Her teachers have been saying that Amy has been dropping out of PE sessions and, on occasion, is rude and difficult in class.

On questioning, it was noted that Amy coughed mainly at night and with exercise. It was also noted that Amy's mum had asthma and also suffered from various allergies. A diagnosis of asthma was therefore very likely; however, it needed to be confirmed.

Amy's peak flow rate at the time was 160 l/min, and her predicted peak flow was 230 l/min. It was decided therefore to do a reversibility test. Amy was given a B2 agonist, and peak flow was measured again 15 minutes later. Amy's peak flow had increased to 220 l/min, an increase of 29 % and 60 l/min. The diagnosis therefore was asthma.

Figure 4.8. Amy's story.

the wheeze is heard on auscultation and clearly distinguishable from upper airway sounds.

Very often, cough will be the only presenting feature, so it is important to find out when the child coughs – for example, is it worse at night or with exercise, or are there any other identifiable factors that make it worse?

Bill's story

Bill is a 57-year-old retired police officer and is married to Emily. They have two grown-up children who are both married. Bill has been fairly fit all his life, but over the last three or four years he has been getting increasingly breathless, especially on exertion. However, he put this down to his age and did not go to the doctor. Over the last winter he had two chest infections which needed treatment with antibiotics. This winter he has already had three chest infections and now feels that he is developing another. He finds that he has great difficulty walking up even the smallest incline, has a productive cough most mornings and is generally finding life quite difficult. Bill smoked from his early teens until he was 35 and his father died from chest disease at the age of 65.

On questioning, it was discovered that Bill generally only had symptoms when doing anything that required any effort. Usually at rest he felt alright, and rarely coughed at night.

Spirometry showed moderate obstruction and there was little reversibility, neither to bronchodilators nor steroids. A chest X-ray showed emphysematous changes. Bill's likely diagnosis was therefore COPD.

Figure 4.9. Bill's story.

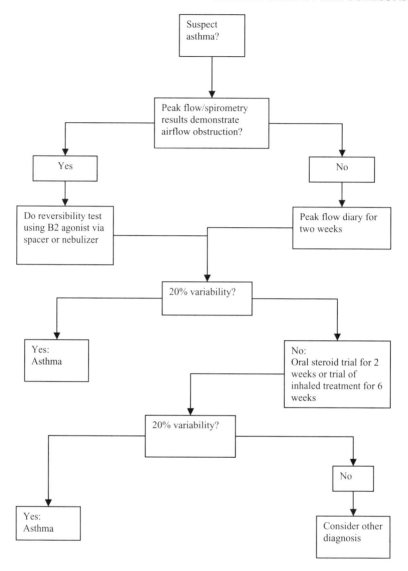

Figure 4.10. Flow chart summarizing the diagnosis of asthma.

The British Thoracic Society Guideline [2] advises that the diagnosis of asthma in young children should be based on the following three criteria:

- the presence of key features and careful consideration of alternative diagnoses;
- assessment of the response to trials of treatment, and ongoing assessment;
- repeated reassessment of the child, questioning the diagnosis if management is ineffective.

Table 4.2. Symptom diary showing typical scores for a child with asthma

Numbers of days	1	2	3	4	5	6	7
Night-time symptoms							
None = 0							
Slight = 1							
Waking 2–3 times = 2	2	3	3	2	2	3	2
Bad night/awake most of night = 3							
Daytime symptoms							
Wheeze: None = 0							
Occasional = 1							
Moderate = 2	1	3	3	2	3	3	2
Severe = 3							
Cough: None = 0							
Occasional = 1							
Frequent = 2	2	2	1	2	1	2	2
Symptoms on exercise							
None = 0							
Running = 1							
Walking = 2	3	2	2	1	2	3	2
Limited activity = 3							
Daily total	8	10	9	7	8	11	8
Number of doses of reliever medication given	3	3	3	2	3	4	2

With children aged two to five years, it is usual to try some therapy and ask the parents to keep a symptom diary to assess any response to the treatment.

Table 4.2 shows an example of a symptom diary kept for a young child. The total daily scores and reliever usage show high levels of symptoms which are suggestive of asthma.

Table 4.3 shows a symptom diary for the same child two weeks after being prescribed an inhaled steroid. Note how the scores gradually improve which indicates that the child is responding to the treatment and therefore has a likely diagnosis of asthma.

When you are finally confident that the patient does have asthma, you can then move on to decide on the most suitable treatment. However, if after taking a thorough clinical history, and obtaining reliable objective measurements of lung function, the diagnosis is not as clear as you would like it to be, you will need to look at other possible reasons for the symptoms. The next section explores other possible diagnoses; however, at this stage it is probably wise to refer to a medical colleague for help with clarifying the diagnosis.

DIFFERENTIAL DIAGNOSES

To be able to give the correct treatment and management, it is essential to get the diagnosis right. This may seem to be stating the obvious, but patients do get

Table 4.3. Symptom diary two weeks after commencing inhaled corticosteroid

Numbers of days	21	22	23	24	25	26	27
Night-time symptoms							
None = 0							
Slight = 1							
Waking 2–3 times = 2	1	1	2	1	0	1	0
Bad night/awake most of night = 3							
Daytime symptoms							
Wheeze: None = 0							
Occasional = 1							
Moderate =2	0	1	1	1	2	1	1
Severe = 3							
Cough: None = 0							
Occasional = 1							
Frequent = 2	1	1	0	1	0	0	0
Symptoms on exercise							
None = 0							
Running = 1							
Walking = 2	2	1	1	0	2	1	1
Limited activity = 3							
Daily total	4	4	4	3	4	3	2
Number of doses of reliever medication given	2	2	2	1	2	1	0

misdiagnosed, or sometimes receive no diagnosis at all! For example, a patient may be told they have asthma when they have COPD, or get diagnosed with recurrent chest infections when they have asthma. However, it is also important not to miss other possible diagnoses. If you are unsure about the diagnosis, do not hesitate to pass it on to someone with more experience, for example the patient's GP or even a hospital consultant.

There are several clues that might make you suspect that perhaps the condition isn't asthma, for example, if there is little or no response to treatment, or the clinical findings don't match the lung function results. When trying to 'tease out' the diagnosis, look again at the family history. For example, did either of the parents or grandparents suffer from any unusual chest complaint, or has a family member died unexpectedly early from a respiratory disease? In any patient where the diagnosis is unclear, or if they have additional unexplained symptoms, it may be useful to do a chest X-ray. Tables 4.4 and 4.5 summarize the indications for referral for specialist opinion and possible other causes for the symptoms.

GASTRO-OESOPHAGEAL REFLUX

Occasionally patients with asthma may also have oesophageal reflux. This is a slightly confusing issue as there is some conflict over whether asthma is triggered by oe-sophageal reflux, or whether oesophageal reflux is triggered by asthma. Treatment is usually with antacids, or drugs that block the production of stomach acid, for

Table 4.4. Indications for referral for specialist opinion

Indications for referral for specialist opinion or further investigation	
• Doubt about the diagnosis	• Unilateral or fixed wheeze
• Unusual clinical findings	• Stridor
• Lung function results do not correspond to the clinical history	• Suspected occupational asthma
• Persistent shortness of breath	• Persistent chest pain
• Persistent cough	• Weight loss
• Persistent sputum production	• Nonresolving chest infection

example proton pump inhibitors. It remains controversial as to whether this has any effect on asthma symptoms, and a recent Cochrane review [3] has found that there was no overall benefit in asthma symptoms following treatment for gastro-oesophageal reflux.

CONGESTIVE CARDIAC FAILURE

This often presents with acute episodes of night-time breathlessness and wheeze. The breathlessness in this case is usually relieved by sitting upright. One clue may be swollen ankles and feet. The clinical and radiological features differ from asthma, but occasionally, right-sided heart failure, or cor pulmonale may develop in some patients with severe chronic asthma or COPD.

CHRONIC OBSTRUCTIVE PULMONARY DISEASE (COPD)

COPD is an umbrella term for diseases such as emphysema and chronic bronchitis. We have already discussed the fact that asthma is a variable lung condition, with fluctuations in lung function and symptoms. COPD, on the other hand, is a fixed airways disease. This means that the damage done to the airways, usually through smoking, is irreversible, even with treatment. It most commonly becomes apparent in people over the age of thirty-five, who are, or who have been smokers.

Table 4.5. Table listing possible differential diagnoses

Possible differential diagnoses	
• Gastro-oesophageal reflux	• Cystic fibrosis
• Congestive cardiac failure	• Interstitial lung disease
• COPD	• Pulmonary emboli
• Alpha-1 antitrypsin deficiency	• Foreign body
• Bronchiectasis	• Aspiration
• Tumour	• Vocal cord dysfunction
• Hyperventilation	• Bronchopulmonary aspergillosis

Occasionally, people who have 'difficult to control' asthma, or who have frequent asthma exacerbations, will go on to develop COPD. This is due to scarring, or fibrosis of the airways leading to loss of elasticity. This is sometimes called airway wall remodelling, which is discussed in more detail in Chapter 3.

There is no single test which can be used to diagnose COPD. Diagnosis is based on effective history-taking, signs and symptoms, and is confirmed with spirometry. The most effective treatment strategy is to stop smoking if the patient has not done so already. This is the only intervention that has been shown to halt the rapid decline in lung function that accompanies this disease. Other treatment strategies are aimed at controlling symptoms, preventing exacerbations and improving quality of life.

ALPHA-1 ANTITRYPSIN DEFICIENCY

Alpha-1 antitrypsin is a protein present in normal lungs and protects lung tissue from being digested by destructive enzymes. Deficiency of alpha-1 antitrypsin results in damage to the lung tissue, which means that enzymes actually digest healthy lung tissue. It is an inherited condition where both parents will carry the gene.

If your asthmatic patient has abnormal lung function, is not responding to treatment and has a family history of abnormal chest disease, you may consider testing for deficiency of alpha-1 antitrypsin. This is done by a blood test which measures levels of alpha-1 antitrypsin. The patient may either be totally deficient, or just have lower levels than normal.

At present there is no effective treatment for alpha-1 antitrypsin deficiency. There have been trials of alpha-1 antitrypsin replacement therapy and this is available in some countries, but not as yet in the UK. The most important aspect in the management of this condition is advice and education about smoking. Genetic counselling is also usually offered to families where alpha-1 antitrypsin deficiency has been diagnosed.

BRONCHIECTASIS

Bronchiectasis is a chronic lung disease characterized by irreversible dilatation of the bronchi. This is usually as a result of inflammation and infection. If there is a local cause, an inhaled foreign body, for example, the condition may be confined to one area of the lung. If, however, there is a more general cause – for example, immunoglobulin deficiency – the condition will be much more diffuse throughout the lungs. Symptoms include cough and excessive sputum production which is often purulent.

Patients who are immunodeficient often present with repeated childhood respiratory infections, but the disease may not be diagnosed until adulthood when bronchiectasis becomes fully established.

LUNG TUMOURS

The pathology of lung cancer is complicated; however, it is broadly classified into two groups:

- small-cell carcinoma which accounts for about 25 % of all lung cancers;
- non-small-cell carcinoma which accounts for 75 % of all lung cancers.

Small-cell carcinoma is highly malignant and grows and metastasizes very quickly, whereas non-small-cell carcinoma is much slower growing with a much better prognosis.

Lung cancers which occur in the larger airways often present with symptoms such as cough, breathlessness and haemoptysis. Peripheral cancers, on the other hand may be present for some time without any symptoms becoming apparent until the disease is well advanced.

HYPERVENTILATION

Hyperventilation, or overbreathing as it is sometimes called, is usually caused by anxiety or panic. The breathing typically becomes rapid and deep and actually makes the patient feel very breathless. It leads to increased levels of oxygen and low levels of carbon dioxide in the blood.

Hyperventilation can be confusing, especially if it occurs in a patient with known asthma. Signs and symptoms include dizziness, shortness of breath, confusion and numbness or tingling in the arms or around the mouth. It can occasionally cause tetany in the hands. If you are in any doubt, particularly if the patient is known to have asthma, it is safer to treat it as asthma rather than delaying possibly life-saving treatment.

CYSTIC FIBROSIS

Cystic fibrosis is an inherited disease caused by an abnormal gene that has to be present in both parents. It affects around 7500 people in the UK. It can affect a number of organs, particularly the lungs and pancreas which become clogged up by thick, sticky mucus. Symptoms include poor weight gain, cough, repeated chest infections, abnormal stools and salty sweat.

There is no cure for cystic fibrosis, but the faulty gene has been identified. With treatment most patients are now living longer and the average life expectancy for someone with the disease is around 31 years.

INTERSTITIAL LUNG DISEASE

There are a number of conditions that affect the interstitial tissue between the alveoli, resulting in fibrosis, or scarring, of the lung tissue. The lung loses its elasticity and becomes very stiff, causing extreme breathlessness. These conditions include

pulmonary fibrosis and fibrosing alveolitis. The symptoms and progression of the disease may vary from person to person. There is very little that can be offered in the way of treatment. Occasionally steroid therapy may be helpful and many patients end up on long-term oxygen therapy.

The cause of interstitial lung disease is unknown, but inhaling environmental pollutants is thought to be a large contributing factor. People who work with asbestos, for example, and farmers and bird-keepers are all at risk from developing the condition. You may hear the terms interstitial lung disease, pulmonary fibrosis or interstitial pulmonary fibrosis, but basically they all mean the same thing.

PULMONARY EMBOLI

A pulmonary embolus is a blockage of an artery in the lungs by a blood clot, fat, air or clumped tumour cells. It is most commonly caused by a deep vein thrombosis which occurs through prolonged inactivity such as bed rest or long aeroplane trips. Other risk factors include oral contraceptive use, childbirth and surgery (especially pelvic surgery). Sometimes a pulmonary embolus will clear up on its own, but occasionally it can cause serious illness and it is occasionally fatal.

The symptoms of pulmonary emboli are usually of sudden onset and include cough, shortness of breath and chest pain. Additional symptoms that may be associated with the condition are wheezing, cyanosis and nasal flaring. Patients will need to be admitted to hospital and receive thrombolytic therapy to dissolve the clot.

FOREIGN BODY

Children have a great knack for being able to insert small objects such as beads or nuts into the smallest orifice, as parents – or indeed anyone who has worked in an accident and emergency (A & E) department – will know.

Larger foreign bodies will lodge in the trachea and cause cough, stridor and possibly cyanosis. The patient will probably be very distressed. Small foreign bodies such as peanuts tend to lodge in the right main bronchus where they cause wheeze and cough. If left for any length of time, there may be hyperinflation on the unaffected side.

If there is a very small inhaled foreign body, it may not be discovered for a long period of time, possibly years after the initial event. This could then lead to chronic lung diseases such as bronchiectasis.

ASPIRATION

Occasionally, an inhaled foreign body leads to aspiration pneumonia. This usually happens when a patient inhales food, drink or vomit into the lungs which become infected with bacteria. Sometimes a lung abscess will form.

Symptoms include fever, cough and sputum production which is usually foul smelling. There will also be breathlessness, wheeze and possibly cyanosis. The patient will need antibiotic therapy and hospital admission may be necessary. Aspiration pneumonia is a serious condition which may be prolonged and can lead to death.

VOCAL CORD DYSFUNCTION

This is an important differential diagnosis in younger patients. There are episodes of semiclosure of the glottis which produces both inspiratory and expiratory wheezes. Symptoms are usually variable and lung function and blood gases are normal. Response to asthma treatment is usually poor.

This condition is often found in patients in whom there is a history of psychiatric or psychological stress. However, it is important to note that occasionally, there is vocal cord dysfunction in an acute asthma attack. These patients should not be considered to have psychogenic asthma.

ALLERGIC BRONCHOPULMONARY ASPERGILLOSIS

Fungal spores containing *Aspergillus fumigatus* are usually found on riverbanks, marshes and forests, or wherever there is wet or decaying vegetation. Other sources include wet paint, construction materials and in air conditioning systems. Around 2–4 % of patients with asthma are thought to be sensitive to these spores and go on to develop allergic bronchopulmonary aspergillosis. In this condition, the fungus colonizes the mucus in the airways and causes recurrent allergic inflammation. In severe cases, this can lead to bronchiectasis.

A diagnosis of bronchopulmonary aspergillosis should be suspected when asthmatic patients present with progressively worsening symptoms of asthma and possibly a mild fever. Chest X-rays often resemble the features of pneumonia, but these features move around on subsequent chest X-rays. The fungus itself may be seen on microscopic examination of the mucus, and blood tests show increased levels of eosinophils and antibodies to Aspergillus.

Treatment is usually with high doses of corticosteroids and bronchodilators. The majority of patients will need oral corticosteroid therapy on a long-term basis, rather than inhaled corticosteroids. Occasionally the antifungal drug itraconazole may help.

SUMMARY

Getting the diagnosis right is fundamental to the management of asthma, and this chapter has stressed the importance of structured assessment, and the objective tests that can be performed to confirm the diagnosis. It is also important to have an understanding of the possible differential diagnoses, and know when to refer the patient for specialist opinion. Once you are sure of the diagnosis, you can move on with confidence to the management of asthma.

REFERENCES

1. British Thoracic Society and Association of Respiratory Technicians and Physiologists (1994) Guidelines for the measurement of respiratory function. *Respiratory Medicine*, **38**, 165–94.
2. British Thoracic Society/Scottish Intercollegiate Guidelines Network (2005) *British Guideline on the Management of Asthma*, Revised edition. Available at www.brit-thoracic.org.uk/guidelines.html.
3. Gibson, P.G., Henry, R.L., Coughlan, J.L. (2006) Gastro-oesophageal reflux treatment for asthma in adults and children. *The Cochrane Database of Systematic Reviews* (4), 1464–780X.

5 Drug Therapy in Asthma

Key points:

- The role of drug therapy in asthma is to reduce inflammation and swelling in the airways, leading to less bronchial hyperreactivity and fewer symptoms.
- The two main types of drug therapy in asthma are known as preventers and relievers.
- The most effective preventers currently available are inhaled corticosteroids.
- The majority of asthma medication is given via the inhaled route, which leads to less side effects.

INTRODUCTION

The aim of asthma management is to control symptoms, prevent exacerbations and achieve best possible lung function. As discussed in Chapter 3, asthma is an inflammatory condition, with subsequent airway narrowing in response to contact with an allergen or other trigger. The role of drug therapy in asthma is to reduce the inflammation and swelling in the airways leading to less bronchial hyperreactivity and therefore less symptoms.

Two main types of treatment are involved in this process and the most simple way to think of them is to divide them into preventers and relievers. As the names suggest, preventers work on the airways to prevent symptoms and relievers are used for relief of symptoms when they occur. The most effective preventers currently in use are corticosteroids. Relievers are bronchodilators which open up the airways. The safest and most effective way of giving both these drugs is via the inhaled route. This means that much lower doses are able to be used, thus reducing the risk of side effects. In addition, because it is going directly to the lungs, the drug has a much quicker onset of action. Oral preparations are also available and will be discussed under each heading.

The goal in the pharmacological management of asthma is to control the condition using the lowest dose of drug possible. In its stepwise approach, the British Thoracic Society [1] advises starting treatment at the step most appropriate to the severity of the patient's asthma. The management of asthma will be addressed in Chapter 7, so the aim of this chapter is to discuss the currently available drugs and how they work.

CORTICOSTEROIDS

Mode of Action

Corticosteroids inhibit the inflammatory process and are the most effective way of controlling asthma symptoms in adults and children. They work by entering target cells and binding to glucocorticoid receptors in the cytoplasm. This combination is then transported to the nucleus where they attach to specific parts of the DNA. This results in increased transcription of anti-inflammatory proteins and decreased transcription of proinflammatory genes. They also inhibit the effects of many of the inflammatory and harmful cells that are activated in an asthma attack. The end result is a reduction in airway hyperreactivity.

Clinical Use

Inhaled corticosteroids are recommended at step 2 of the BTS Clinical Guideline [1], for both adults and children. Oral corticosteroids are reserved for the management of acute asthma, and occasionally on a long-term basis for patients at step 5 of the Guideline [1], whose asthma is difficult to control on other therapies. A list of the most commonly used inhaled steroids is given in Table 5.1.

INHALED CORTICOSTEROIDS

In clinical practice beclometasone and budesonide are approximately equivalent in dosages; however, there may be small variations with different delivery devices. Fluticasone is equivalent to beclometasone and budesonide at half the dosage. QVAR is a form of beclometasone which, similar to fluticasone, should be given at half the dose of normal beclometasone.

Early studies suggest that the two newer inhaled corticosteroids, mometasone and ciclesonide may be equipotent with fluticasone, but at present, the evidence is not fully substantiated.

A proportion of all currently available inhaled corticosteroids are systemically absorbed from the lungs, but the extent of systemic absorption is dependent on

Table 5.1. Currently available inhaled corticosteroids

Generic name	Brand name
Beclometasone dipropionate	Beclazone
	QVAR
	Aerobec
	Asmabec
	Clenil Modulite
Budesonide	Pulmicort
Fluticasone	Flixotide
Mometasone furoate	Asmanex
Ciclesonide	Alvesco

several factors such as inhaler device and particle size. The speed at which systemic absorption takes place is also dependent on factors such as the choice of drug. Fluticasone, for example, is very slowly absorbed compared with beclometasone or budesonide.

A large proportion of the drug will also be swallowed and absorbed from the gut where again it will enter the systemic circulation. The amount of drug swallowed and absorbed in this way will depend on the type of delivery device used, inhaler technique and whether a spacer device is utilized.

Dose of Inhaled Steroids

In deciding on the dose of inhaled corticosteroid, remember that the aim of treatment is to control symptoms using as low a dose as possible. In children, 200 mcg a day of beclometasone (or equivalent) is usually sufficient to control symptoms, and in adults, 400 mcg a day of beclometasone (or equivalent). However, you should always refer to clinical guidelines as appropriate.

Inhaled steroids are usually given twice a day. There is some evidence that once daily dosing, particularly with the newer inhaled corticosteroid ciclesonide, may be sufficient in controlling asthma. The problem with this is that patients do occasionally forget to take their medication which could be a problem in a once daily regime. There is no evidence that taking inhaled steroids more than twice a day confers any benefit. The dosage of inhaled steroids will be dealt with in more detail in Chapter 7 on the management of asthma.

Length of Action

Inhaled steroids take approximately two weeks to reach their full effect and it may take up to a month before there is any significant preventative effect on asthma symptoms. This is the reason that inhaled steroids have to be taken on a daily basis in order to do their job of reducing inflammation and preventing the subsequent airway narrowing that occurs in asthma.

Quite often patients will think that the treatment is not working and stop taking it, or take it on a haphazard basis. It is important therefore to explain that they will probably not experience any substantial reduction in their symptoms for several weeks and that they should persevere with the treatment. Similarly, when patients are established on inhaled steroid therapy, they frequently do not understand the importance of taking it regularly every day when they are not experiencing any symptoms. Education and explanation is therefore vitally important when managing the patient with asthma and will be discussed in more detail in Chapter 7.

Choice of Inhaled Steroid

The choice of inhaled corticosteroid will depend on considerations such as the severity of symptoms together with the availability of an inhaler device, and the ability and willingness of the patient to use it. An inhaler which the patient will and can use is obviously going to work much better than an inhaler that is either not being used properly or left in a cupboard because the patient does not like it. Local guidelines and formularies may limit the choice available to the practitioner.

Side Effects of Inhaled Corticosteroids

In normal recommended daily doses, inhaled steroids do not usually pose too much of a problem as regards side effects. Because the drug is being inhaled, it has the advantage of being used in much smaller doses, therefore with less risk of side effects. However, even with good inhaler technique, a proportion of the drug will be systemically absorbed.

The side effects from inhaled steroids are usually minimal and mainly localized to the mouth and oropharynx. Patients sometimes complain of oral candidiasis, sore throat and hoarse voice. These effects can be minimized by using a spacer device with a metered dose inhaler and rinsing the mouth out after using an inhaled steroid. Antifungal treatment may help if this becomes a problem.

Corticosteroids inhibit the body's natural production of cortisol by a negative feedback on the pituitary gland. In simple terms this means that the pituitary gland becomes aware that cortisol is being obtained from another source and therefore either shuts down or decreases production. This process is known as adrenal suppression and is dose dependent, most often occurring when more than 10 mg prednisolone is used daily. Adrenal suppression can also occur when using high doses of inhaled corticosteroids, say more than 1500 mcg of beclometasone (or equivalent) a day in adults and 800 mcg of beclometasone (or equivalent) a day in children. This is a very serious side effect of corticosteroids and very often patients will need hospital treatment to recover. Total recovery can take many months. Signs and symptoms of adrenal suppression include weight loss, fatigue, nausea and weakness. These symptoms are usually insidious and come on over a long period of time, so it may be difficult to attribute them to inhaled steroid use.

Occasionally patients who are using high doses of inhaled steroids to control their asthma will have a short synacthen test done to assess their adrenal reserve. Synacthen is tetracosactrin, one of the amino acids of adrenocorticotrophic hormone (ACTH). After taking a blood sample to measure baseline cortisol levels, synacthen is given intravenously or intramuscularly. Further blood samples are then taken at 30 and 60 min. In normal health, the baseline plasma cortisol should rise from about 170 mmol/l to at least 580 mmol/l. The patient with adrenal suppression will be unable to raise their cortisol level in response to synacthen.

There have been concerns about growth retardation in children when using higher doses of inhaled steroids. More recent studies have shown that eventual height is usually normal; however, parents of children will need explanation and reassurance about this issue. There is also an increased risk of bone fracture and cataracts in elderly patients.

Table 5.2. Currently available oral corticosteroids

Generic name	Brand name
Prednisolone	Deltacortril

Inhaled corticosteroids have revolutionized asthma management over the last thirty years, and have been shown to reduce the numbers of acute episodes, and therefore the need for oral corticosteroids. The associated risks must therefore be taken into context with their beneficial effects. The important message is to use the lowest dose possible to control the asthma, and to use a spacer device to reduce oropharyngeal deposition.

ORAL CORTICOSTEROIDS

Oral corticosteroids are used to treat an acute exacerbation of asthma, and occasionally on a long-term basis for difficult to control asthma. The currently available oral corticosteroids are shown in Table 5.2. Prednisolone takes approximately six hours to work, so it is important that it is given as early as possible in an acute asthma attack.

A course of oral corticosteroids usually lasts for five to seven days for adults. Because of concerns about adrenal suppression, in the past the dose of oral corticosteroids was always tapered off to give the body a chance to restart its own production of cortisol. However, this is now considered to be unnecessary and following an acute exacerbation, oral steroids can be stopped abruptly and do not need to be tapered as long as the patient is receiving an adequate dose of inhaled steroid. In rare instances where oral steroids have to be given for longer than three weeks, or the patient is on maintenance oral steroid therapy, the dose should be tapered off.

Side Effects of Oral Corticosteroids

Oral steroids are very effective in the management of acute asthma and occasionally as maintenance therapy in difficult to control asthma. Given as a short course following an acute exacerbation, usually 40 mg a day for five to seven days in adults, or 20–30 mg a day for three days in children, there are usually no problems with side effects. (The dose of prednisolone for acute asthma attacks will be dealt with in more detail in Chapter 9.)

In patients on maintenance therapy and those who have recurrent acute attacks, therefore having frequent courses of oral steroids, there is more of a risk of side effects. As discussed before, probably the most important side effect is adrenal suppression. There is, however, a whole list of other possible unwanted side effects with oral corticosteroid therapy. Unfortunately, many of these side effects are permanent and even when the patient stops taking oral corticosteroids, some of them, such as thinning of the bones and skin, will remain. The side effects of oral corticosteroids are listed below:

- Osteoporosis
- Thinning of the skin
- Bruising
- Mood changes
- Precipitation of diabetes
- Growth retardation
- Moon face

- Masking of infection
- Peptic ulceration
- Weight gain
- Oedema
- Hypertension and cardiac failure
- Delayed wound healing
- Cataracts

Again, as with inhaled corticosteroid therapy, it is important to weigh up the risks and benefits. At the present time, oral corticosteroids are the only effective treatment for acute asthma and should be given as early as possible in the acute attack.

Intramuscular/Intravenous Corticosteroids

Intramuscular or intravenous corticosteroids, usually hydrocortisone, are used in the management of acute asthma only when the patient is unable to swallow because of vomiting or if unconscious. The length of action is similar to oral corticosteroids, so there is no advantage to using it instead of prednisolone.

BRONCHODILATORS

Inhaled bronchodilators fall into two categories:

- B2 agonists
- anticholinergics

Both open up the airways but work in different ways. In order to understand the way they work, you will need to remind yourself of the workings of the central nervous system which was described in Chapter 2. If you remember, the central nervous system is divided into two: the autonomic nervous system which is involuntary and the somatic nervous system which is voluntary. The respiratory system is largely controlled by the involuntary autonomic nervous system, and many drugs act on this system.

The autonomic nervous system is further divided into the sympathetic and parasympathetic nervous system. The sympathetic nervous system is responsible for the production of adrenaline, which you will probably have heard of as the fight or flight hormone. It is in fact a chemical messenger, which crosses over the gap, or synapse, between the nerve ending and the target tissue. When the body comes under stress, either from a frightening situation or stressful circumstances, adrenaline pours into the bloodstream, raising the blood pressure and increasing the pulse rate, allowing

Table 5.3. Currently available short-acting bronchodilators

Generic name	Brand name
Salbutamol	Ventolin
	Salamol
	Airomir
	Pulvinal
	Asmasal
	Volmax (tablets)
Terbutaline	Bricanyl

you to either put up a fight and cope with the situation, or run away. The increased adrenaline also combines with beta 2 receptors in the smooth muscle in the airway walls, relaxing the muscle and opening up the airways.

Bronchodilating drugs such as salbutamol imitate this action, and you may sometimes hear them called sympathomimetics for this reason. When inhaled they target the B2 receptors in the bronchial smooth muscle leading to muscle relaxation and subsequent widening of the airways, or bronchodilatation. They are also known as B2 agonists, B2 stimulants or adrenergics. In the management of asthma there are two types of B2 agonist available:

- Short-acting B2 agonists are used for quick relief of symptoms or to prevent exercise-induced asthma.
- Long-acting B2 agonists are used regularly on a twice-a-day basis to help control symptoms, improve lung function and prevent exacerbations.

We shall concentrate on the short-acting inhaled B2 agonists first, and these are listed in Table 5.3.

Short-Acting Inhaled B2 Agonists

These drugs are used for relief of symptoms when they have started and are also effective at controlling exercise-induced asthma if taken 15–30 min prior to exercise. The British Thoracic Society's Guideline [1] in its stepwise approach, recommends that an inhaled short-acting B2 agonist should be used when required at step 1 for mild, intermittent asthma.

B2 agonists are also available in injection form, but their use is specialized and should only be considered when the patient is being managed by a respiratory consultant. Oral formulations are also available, but are generally not recommended because they are not so effective and there is a greater risk of side effects. They should be reserved for the small minority of patients who are unable to use inhalers.

Table 5.4. Currently available long-acting bronchodilators

Generic name	Brand name
Salmeterol	Serevent
Formoterol	Oxis
	Atimos
	Foradil

Long-Acting B2 Agonists (LABA)

Long-acting B2 agonists are used as an add-on therapy to inhaled corticosteroids at step 3 of the BTS Clinical Guideline, and are used twice a day on a regular basis. The ones currently in use are listed in Table 5.4. They work in a similar way to the short-acting versions but have exceptional binding to the B2 receptors resulting in a long-acting action of up to 12 h. They are extremely effective in controlling symptoms and preventing exacerbations. Salmeterol takes approximately 30 min to start to have any effect, so it should not be used in the treatment of an acute asthma attack. Formoterol has a slightly faster onset of action, but again is not recommended in acute asthma.

Side Effects of Inhaled B2 Agonists

Inhaled B2 agonists are very safe drugs with minimal side effects if used at the recommended dosage. If you remember, they combine with B2 receptors in the bronchial smooth muscle to produce bronchodilatation. However, Beta 2 receptors can also be found in skeletal and heart muscle, and the drug will also find its way to these parts of the body. The side effects of B2 agonists, therefore, are the result of stimulation of receptors outside the lungs, for example, fine tremor because of its effect on B2 receptors in skeletal muscle and tachycardia as a result of its effect on cardiac muscle. Other side effects of B2 agonists include headaches and muscle cramp. Occasionally there is a risk of hypokalaemia when high doses of B2 agonists are used.

Over the last 30–40 years there has been a great debate as to whether the use of B2 agonist drugs has contributed to asthma deaths. In the mid 1960s, for example, there was a sharp rise and subsequent fall in asthma deaths in several countries, including the United Kingdom, which was linked to the introduction of isoprenaline, a nonselective B agonist drug. The death rate fell when the drug was subsequently withdrawn. In New Zealand in the 1970s an increase in asthma deaths corresponded to an increase in prescriptions for another B2 agonist, fenoterol.

Three recent studies [2–4] found that there was high usage of short-acting bronchodilators among patients who died from asthma, but the authors could not conclude whether the drugs actually contributed to these deaths. It has been suggested that patients with severe disease would naturally be using more short-acting bronchodilators,

Table 5.5. Currently available anticholinergics

Generic name	Brand name
Ipratropium bromide	Atrovent
Tiotropium bromide	Spiriva

and that it was the severity of the disease rather than the drugs that actually caused the deaths.

In 2006, the results of a large American study were published investigating asthma deaths in relation to the use of long-acting B2 agonists. This study concluded that there were more asthma deaths in the group of patients using a long-acting B2 agonist than in the placebo group [5]. However, the majority of the patients who died were not using an inhaled steroid, and were from a more disadvantaged social background. Similarly, a meta-analysis of studies looking at long-acting B2 agonist use and asthma severity found that those patients using these drugs had a higher hospital admission rate and episodes of life-threatening asthma [6]. However, there has been some debate as to the interpretation of the data of this particular study. In contrast to both these studies, researchers in the UK found that there was no connection between asthma deaths and the use of long-acting B2 agonists [7]. The Commission on Human Medicines has now recommended that further, reliable research is conducted into this issue.

Recommendations for the Use of Long-Acting B2 Agonists

Despite the controversies surrounding the use of long-acting B2 agonists, it is still considered that the benefits far outweigh the risks, and that clinicians should carry on using them. The Medicines and Healthcare products Regulation Agency (MHRA), however, which is an executive agency of the Department of Health, has issued guidelines for their use which are summarized in Chapter 7.

ANTICHOLINERGICS

Anticholinergics, sometimes called antimuscarinic bronchodilators, are shown in Table 5.5. They act on the parasympathetic nervous system. The chemical messenger in this case is acetylcholine. When an irritant such as smoke or dust is inhaled, the brain sends out a message which passes along the nerve and is carried by acetylcholine across the gap or synapse, to combine with cholinergic receptors in the bronchial smooth muscle to cause the muscle to constrict, thus narrowing the airways. This is a protective mechanism which also triggers the cough reflex. In patients with asthma this reaction may be highly exaggerated and could lead to an acute asthma attack.

This bronchoconstricting effect is obviously opposite to the result you need when treating the patient with asthma. Therefore the process needs to be prevented or blocked. Ipratropium is an anticholinergic drug which works by blocking the action of the parasympathetic nervous system and preventing the airways constricting. There are two types of anticholinergic drug available:

- Short-acting anticholinergics are used three to four times a day to help control the symptoms of chronic obstructive pulmonary disease (COPD), or problematic asthma, that is difficult to control. They are also used in the management of acute asthma.
- Long-acting anticholinergics are used regularly once a day to help control the symptoms of COPD.

Clinical Use

Anticholinergic drugs are not recommended in the day-to-day management of asthma, but occasionally in patients with difficult to control asthma they may be used as an add-on therapy. They have also been shown to be effective in treating an acute exacerbation when given in addition to a B2 agonist, and are recommended in acute severe, or life-threatening asthma.

Occasionally, in very young children anticholinergic drugs are more effective in relieving airway narrowing than B2 agonists. This is thought to be because the B2 receptors in bronchial smooth muscle are not terribly well developed until the child is between two and three years of age. In patients with COPD, an anticholinergic is often more effective than B2 agonists.

Length of Action

Ipratropium has a fairly slow onset of action and takes 30–40 min to take effect and lasts for 4–6 h. Tiotropium is a recently introduced long-acting anticholinergic drug which is given once a day. It is licensed for the management of COPD, and does not have any role at present in treating asthma.

Side Effects of Anticholinergics

Anticholinergic drugs have very little side effects because there is almost no systemic absorption. There have been reports of paradoxical bronchospasm when nebulizing with ipratropium, but this is rare and is thought to have been the result of the components of an earlier nebulizer solution.

In elderly patients there is a risk of glaucoma when nebulizing with ipratropium due to the mist formed from the nebulization process coming into direct contact with the eye. This can be avoided by using a mouthpiece rather than a mask. Other possible side effects are dry mouth, constipation and blurred vision.

To summarize:

- B2 agonists open up the airways by combining with B2 receptors in the bronchial smooth muscle to produce bronchodilatation.
- Anticholinergics prevent the airways constricting by blocking the action of cholinergic receptors in the bronchial smooth muscle.

Table 5.6. Currently available methylxanthines

Generic name	Brand name
Theophylline	Nuelin
	Slo-phyllin
	Uniphyllin
Aminophylline	Phyllocontin

METHYLXANTHINES

This group of drugs are given orally and act as bronchodilators and the drugs most commonly used are listed in Table 5.6. They are also thought to have some anti-inflammatory action as well. Their mode of action is not fully understood, and their bronchodilating effect is more likely to be as a result of combining with other therapies such as inhaled corticosteroids and bronchodilators. In the past they were widely used but because of potential side effects, and the introduction of more efficient, safer forms of therapy, their use has declined.

Methylxanthines, also known as theophyllines, are readily absorbed from the gastro-intestinal tract, but there are problems with maintaining plasma levels which lead to an increased risk of side effects. The drugs work within a narrow therapeutic window, below which there will be no therapeutic effect and above which they become toxic. Optimum plasma concentrations should be between 10 and 20 mg/l.

There are a number of factors which will influence the absorption of the drug. The elderly, for example, have a slower metabolic rate, therefore clearance will be slower than in the young where the metabolic rate is faster. Certain diseases will affect absorption, such as heart disease or hepatic impairment. Methylxanthines will interact with many different drugs, some of which are quite commonly used such as erythromycin or cimetidine. Another problem with methylxanthines is that different brands of the drug can have different absorption rates, so when a patient is established on a particular type of theophylline, it is important that they continue to use the same brand.

Clinical Use

Methylxanthines are recommended as a possible add-on therapy at step 3 of the BTS Clinical Guideline [1], when other therapies are not relieving symptoms. They may also be useful in the treatment of acute severe asthma when they can be given by very slow intravenous infusion.

If you decide to use theophylline in the management of asthma it is important to refer to the guidelines and manufacturer's advice before prescribing.

Side Effects of Methylxanthines

As mentioned before, it is important to maintain plasma concentrations of theophylline inside the therapeutic window. Above this window, side effects will occur and the intensity of the side effects is dose dependent. Gradually increasing the dose until therapeutic concentrations are achieved may reduce the severity of side effects which are listed below:

- Nausea and vomiting
- Headaches
- Tachycardia and/or arrhythmias
- Insomnia
- Convulsions
- Behavioural problems/restlessness
- Gastric problems

Caution

Particular care needs to be taken in the acute situation, as if the patient is already taking a maintenance dose of oral theophylline and an intravenous dose is administered, it could prove fatal.

LEUKOTRIENE RECEPTOR ANTAGONISTS

Cysteinyl-leukotrienes are inflammatory molecules released by mast cells during an asthma attack. They are largely responsible for the bronchoconstriction that occurs during these episodes. They also attract eosinophils into the bronchioles, and it is these eosinophils which not only play a major part in the general hyperresponsiveness of the airways, but also themselves go on to produce more leukotrienes. They are thus responsible for both triggering asthma attacks and also playing a part in long-term hypersensitivity of the airways in chronic, more difficult to control asthma.

   Cysteinyl-leukotrienes are produced from arachidonic acid and cause bronchoconstriction, oedema and also stimulate airway mucus secretion. The action of antileukotrienes therefore is to block this action by preventing leukotriene release from mast cells and eosinophils. They also block the leukotriene receptors in the airways, preventing bronchoconstriction, mucus secretion and oedema. The two currently available leukotriene receptor antagonists are shown in Table 5.7.

Clinical Use

The drug is given orally as a daily add-on therapy at step 3 of the BTS Clinical Guideline [1]. Montelukast is given once daily and Zafirlukast is given twice daily. They have no effect on an acute attack of asthma.

Table 5.7. Currently available leukotriene receptor antagonists

Generic name	Brand name
Montelukast	Singulair
Zafirlukast	Accolate

The difficulty with antileukotriene therapy is that not everyone will benefit from it, and there is no way to predict who will respond best to the treatment. The consensus of opinion seems to be that if there has been no improvement in symptom control after six weeks' treatment, it should be stopped. Patients whose asthma is triggered by aspirin, and who have an allergic component to their asthma, may respond to antileukotriene therapy.

Side Effects of Leukotriene Receptor Antagonists

The most common side effects include gastrointestinal problems and headaches. Rarely, Churg–Strauss syndrome has been reported, characterized by systemic vasculitis and eosinophilia, but in the episodes that have been reported, this unwanted effect was thought to have been precipitated by the withdrawal of oral corticosteroid therapy.

CROMONES

Cromones inhibit various inflammatory cells that play a part in allergic inflammation, including macrophages and eosinophils. They also help to stabilize mast cells in the degranulation process described in Chapter 2. The two drugs that are available are shown in Table 5.8.

Clinical Use

Cromones are a preventative therapy and must be taken regularly. Their disadvantage is that they must be taken 3–4 times a day to be effective, and it generally takes six weeks before any benefit is noticed.

They are sometimes of use in patients who have exercise-induced asthma and have an allergic component to their asthma. However, when compared with inhaled steroids, their use is limited in the modern management of asthma. They do have the great advantage, however, of being nonsteroidal and therefore they are frequently preferred by those patients who are steroid phobic.

Side Effects of Cromone Therapy

Side effects from using cromone therapy are extremely rare. Unfortunately, the inhaled medication does have an unpleasant taste which may affect its use, particularly in children.

Table 5.8. Currently available cromones

Generic name	Brand name
Sodium cromoglycate	Intal
Nedocromil sodium	Tilade

Table 5.9. Currently available combined therapies

Generic components	Brand name
Fluticasone propionate and Salmeterol	Seretide
Budesonide and Formoterol	Symbicort
Salbutamol and Ipratropium bromide	Combivent

COMBINED THERAPIES

Combined therapy inhalers are useful for those patients in whom concordance is an issue. They are also useful for elderly patients, or patients who find it difficult to remember which inhaler they should be taking, and when. The most commonly used combined therapy drugs are shown in Table 5.9. Both Seretide and Symbicort comprise an inhaled steroid and long-acting bronchodilator. There is also a suggestion that the two therapies in one inhaler seem to have beneficial effects over the separate components alone; however, more research needs to be done in this area.

Combivent is a combination of two bronchodilators, a B2 agonist and anticholinergic, which is more often used in COPD.

OTHER THERAPIES

Occasionally people with asthma have very severe, chronic symptoms that do not respond to conventional asthma therapy. These patients will probably be under the care of a respiratory physician and may need further, more aggressive treatment such as immunosuppressant drugs, or anti-IgE therapy. These drugs, and other therapies are discussed in Chapter 10.

SUMMARY

This chapter has discussed all the most commonly used medications in the management of asthma, but pharmaceutical companies are constantly testing new therapies, so newer, perhaps more effective, treatments may become available at any time. It is important to keep up to date with developments in this area, and to be sure of the evidence base and reliability of any new drug before you consider using it for your asthmatic patients.

The mode of action of the drugs has been explained as simply as possible, together with the potential side effects. When deciding on a drug regime for your patient, remember there are many factors to take into consideration such as age, understanding and patient preference. There may also be other issues such as coexisting conditions, allergies and cost. It is important therefore to refer to clinical guidelines where available and also the data sheet for each drug.

Nurses who have undertaken the relevant training are now able to prescribe from the whole British National Formulary, bringing with it many more opportunities for nurses to manage the patient with asthma without referring to a medical colleague. This advancement, however, also brings responsibilities. It is important for all nurse prescribers that they are able to access a forum in their area of work to support clinical governance, and that a structure is in place to enable their continuing professional development.

REFERENCES

1. British Thoracic Society/Scottish Intercollegiate Guidelines Network (2005) *British Guideline on the Management of Asthma*, Revised edition. Available at www.brit-thoracic.org.uk.
2. Anderson, H.R., Ayres, J.G., Sturdy, P.M., *et al.* (2005) Bronchodilator treatment and deaths from asthma: case-control study. *British Medical Journal* **330**, 117–23.
3. Lanes, S.F., Birman, B., Raiford, D., Walker, A.M. (1997) International trends in sales of inhaled fenoterol, all inhaled beta-agonists, and asthma mortality, 1970–1992. *Journal of Clinical Epidemiology* **50** (3), 321–8.
4. Garrett, J.E., Lanes, S.F., Kolbe, J., Rea, H.H. (1996) Risk of severe life threatening asthma and beta agonist type: an example of confounding by severity. *Thorax* **51** (11), 1093–9.
5. Nelson, H.S., Weiss, S.T., Bleeker, E.R. *et al.* (2006) The salmeterol multicenter asthma research trial. A comparison of usual pharmacotherapy for asthma or usual pharmacotherapy plus salmeterol. *Chest* **129**, 15–26.
6. Salpeter, S.R., Buckley, N.S., Ormiston, T.M., Salpeter, E.E. (2006) Meta-analysis: Effect of long-acting B-agonists on severe asthma exacerbations and asthma-related deaths. *Annals of Internal Medicine* **144** (Iss 12).
7. Ross Anderson, H., Ayres, J.G., Sturdy, P.M., *et al.* (2005) Bronchodilator treatment and deaths from asthma: case-control study. *British Medical Journal* **330**, 117.

FURTHER READING

British National Formulary (2006, September) Published by BMJ Publishing Group Ltd. Tavistock Square, London.

6 Inhaler Devices and Nebulizers

Key points:

- Correct inhaler technique is vital to the good management of asthma.
- It is important to ensure that the patient can and will use their inhaler.
- The metered dose inhaler is the most commonly prescribed inhaler, but is the most difficult to use correctly.
- CFC containing metered dose inhalers are gradually being replaced with non-CFC inhalers.
- It is important to inform patients that the new CFC-free metered dose inhalers will feel and taste different from the CFC metered dose inhalers.
- Spacer devices and inhalers must be compatible to provide effective treatment.
- Nebulizers are used to deliver high-dose inhaled drugs in the management of acute asthma.
- It is not recommended for patients with asthma to keep a nebulizer at home for use in an acute attack.

INTRODUCTION

Asthma is a disease of the lungs and therefore it makes much more sense to aim drugs directly at this area, rather than having them travelling around the body before they reach their target site. For this reason, the majority of asthma medication is given via the inhaled route, leading to a more rapid onset of action, and because smaller doses are able to be used, there is less risk of side effects.

However, there are disadvantages to using the inhaled route for medications. Inhalers can be very difficult to use and if inhaler technique is less than perfect, there will be variations in the dose received and subsequently a possible increase in symptoms. This inevitably leads to more hospital admissions and increased use of oral corticosteroids, with the resulting risk of systemic side effects.

This chapter discusses the issues surrounding the choice of inhaler, and describes some of the more commonly used devices.

CHOICE OF DEVICE

When an inhaler is triggered into the mouth, either from an aerosol or dry powder device, the particles released have to be small enough to penetrate deep into the lungs.

The optimal size is less than five microns in diameter. The smaller the particle size, the greater the lung deposition will be. This then seems obvious – we give our patient the inhaler with the smallest particle size for the best symptom control. Unfortunately, it is not as simple as this. Many factors will influence drug delivery, to say nothing about patients' likes and dislikes. Coordination, inspiratory flow rates and extent of obstruction all have a part to play in the success of any chosen device, but perhaps most importantly of all, the patient himself plays the key role in this aspect of asthma management. No matter how efficient the inhaler, or the drugs that are in it, it will not work if the patient cannot or will not use it!

There are a huge number of inhaler devices on the market, and it can sometimes be difficult to make a decision on the most suitable type of device for your patient. Obviously you need to ensure that you are providing an effective, cost-efficient method of drug delivery, but sometimes other considerations have to be taken into account. It is important to assess your patient and decide on the best option: an inhaler which the patient is using correctly, and is subsequently more effective, or an inhaler which is either being used incorrectly, or left in a drawer because the patient does not like it.

With the exception of a small minority, most inhaled drugs come with a choice of devices. Within that choice, there will also be cost implications, and the temptation may be to opt for the cheapest option. The danger of this is that you may be giving the patient a device which they will not or cannot use, leading to the possibility of worsening asthma control. A hospital admission is far more costly than the most expensive inhaler, to say nothing of the distress caused to the patient because of poorly controlled asthma.

The inhaler devices currently in use come in either an aerosol or dry powder format and the choice will depend on a number of issues. Very young children, for example, will not be able to use a dry powder device, and so the only option is to use a metered dose inhaler with spacer. The choice of spacer device is discussed further on in this chapter. Other considerations include the patient's level of understanding, and manual dexterity. Elderly patients with arthritic fingers, or poor eyesight, may find some devices more difficult than others.

Different inhaler devices require varying degrees of inspiratory effort in order to deliver the correct dose of drug into the lungs. A Turbohaler, for example, requires less effort to inhale the medication than a breath-actuated metered dose inhaler. Sometimes there is the concern that the patient's inspiratory capacity is insufficient for the chosen device. To help overcome this problem, several companies have produced an inspiratory flow meter, which measures the patient's inspiratory flow rate and then gives a guide as to the most suitable device depending on the result. Although this may be helpful as a guide in some circumstances, remember that patients are individuals, and there will be other issues that need to be taken into account.

Another point to remember is to check any other inhalers the patient may be using. It is not unknown for a patient to be using three or four different inhaler devices, when all their medication may be available in the same type of inhaler. For example, the patient may be using a metered dose steroid inhaler, a dry powder long-acting B2

> **Issues to consider when deciding on an inhaler device for your patient**
>
> - Ability to use the device
> - Availability of the chosen drug in that device
> - Ability to count the doses remaining
> - Any other inhalers the patient may be using
> - The patient's preference and willingness to use the device
> - Compatibility of inhaler device with spacer

Figure 6.1. Implications and issues surrounding the choice of inhaler device.

agonist, and a breath-actuated reliever inhaler. All these medications could be given either by a metered dose inhaler or dry powder device. The advice is: 'keep it simple'.

Figure 6.1 is a summary of the implications and issues surrounding the choice of inhaler device.

TEACHING CORRECT INHALER TECHNIQUE

As already discussed, correct inhaler technique is vital to the good management of asthma. The choice of device will depend on various issues as described in the previous section of this chapter. It is useful to have a selection of placebo devices to be able to show the patient, so that they can see how they look and feel. It is important to demonstrate the correct use, and then check that the patient has understood and is able to use the chosen inhaler. If you do use placebo devices, however, infection control measures must be in place to protect the patient from coming into contact with bacteria or viruses from contaminated equipment. There are national guidelines available for the care of placebo devices and spacers [1], and each trust or healthcare organization should have a policy for the use and cleaning of placebo inhalers. If you work in general practice, there should be a practice protocol for the cleansing and decontaminating of devices. If there isn't one, perhaps you should consider developing one yourself, in consultation with the GPs and practice manager.

If you are conducting a review of the patient, and he/she is already using inhalers, it is better to ask them to bring their inhalers with them to clinic.

> Inhaler technique should be checked at every opportunity, as it is well known that patients become less competent over time, and will need constant reminding.

The following is a description of the most commonly used devices currently available and the drugs that are available in them. Do not forget, however, that this field of asthma care is constantly changing, so it is important to keep up to date with the latest developments and guidelines.

Table 6.1. Drugs available in metered dose inhalers

Inhaled steroids	B2 Agonists	Anticholinergics	Combined drugs	Others
Beclometasone	Salbutamol	Ipratropium	Seretide	Sodium cromoglycate
Budesonide	Terbutaline		Combivent	Nedocromil sodium
Fluticasone	Salmeterol			
Ciclesonide				

METERED DOSE INHALER

Table 6.1 lists the drugs that are currently available in a metered dose inhaler. The metered dose inhaler is the oldest inhaler on the market and has been available since the early 1950s. The drug is contained in a pressurized aerosol and is mixed with a propellant which helps to propel the drug out of the inhaler and into the mouth and lungs. Each actuation of the device releases a 'metered dose'.

Many drugs are available in this format, and it is probably the most commonly prescribed inhaler. This may be because it is generally cheaper than other devices, but it should be recognized that it is also the most difficult inhaler to use correctly. The main problems are not shaking the device, lack of coordination between pressing the canister and breathing in, and being unable to hold the breath following the inhalation. Even when used accurately, only about 10 % of the medication actually reaches the lungs. The rest is deposited in the mouth and oropharynx, where it is swallowed and may be absorbed from the gastro-intestinal tract.

It is thought that at least 25 % of patients are unable to use a metered dose inhaler correctly, and this figure gets worse with advancing age. Problems with technique are often compounded in the elderly because of problems with manual dexterity, perhaps due to arthritis or other mobility problems. In this case a device called a Haleraid, illustrated in Figure 6.2 may help, which although not available on prescription is quite cheap to buy.

Another problem frequently encountered with metered dose inhalers is the 'cold freon effect' which results from the impact of the aerosol on the back of the throat. This occasionally causes gagging, or coughing, leading to a smaller amount of the drug being deposited in the lungs. In this case, using a spacer may overcome the problem, or it may be necessary to change the device to a dry powder inhaler.

Patients often have difficulty in recognizing when a metered dose inhaler is empty, although the newer CFC-free versions actually stop working when there is nothing left in them. Some metered dose inhalers are now available with a dose counter. It is usually possible to tell how full or empty they are by shaking, but for some patients this can be a problem.

It is important to be aware that towards the end of 2007, some metered dose inhalers are to be withdrawn in order to conform to the laws governing the use of chlorofluorocarbons (CFCs). This will probably affect the availability of beclometasone in its branded form of Becotide and Becloforte in particular, but others may also be

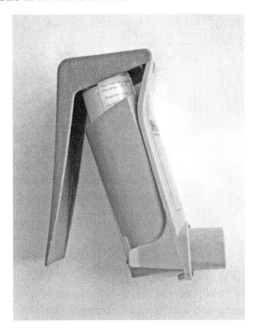

Figure 6.2. Metered dose inhaler with Haleraid.

discontinued as further non-CFC products become more widely available. Patients may be concerned to find that their usual drug therapy is to be changed, therefore it is important to ensure that they understand the reasons for the changeover, and receive extra support and monitoring during the transition period.

Figure 6.3 outlines the correct technique for using a metered dose inhaler.

Inhalation technique for a metered dose inhaler	
• Shake the canister • Breathe out • Put mouthpiece in the mouth • Press the canister and breathe in slowly and deeply • Hold the breath for ten seconds • Breathe out slowly • Wait thirty seconds before repeating	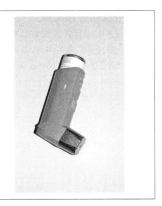

Figure 6.3. Inhalation technique for a metered dose inhaler.

Table 6.2. Drugs available in
the Autohaler device

Inhaled steroids	B2 Agonists
Beclometasone	Salbutamol

BREATH-ACTUATED METERED DOSE INHALER

Using a breath-actuated inhaler overcomes the problem of coordination in pressing
the canister and taking a breath in. These devices are triggered by the patient's
inspiration and respond to quite a low level of inspiratory flow rate. The two devices
available are the Autohaler and the Easi-Breathe. Tables 6.2 and 6.3 list the drugs
that are available in these devices, and Figures 6.4 and 6.5 describe the technique for
using the inhalers.

CHLOROFLUOROCARBONS (CFCs)

Both the manually operated, and the breath-actuated metered dose inhalers contain
a propellant which carries the drug from the inhaler to the lung. This propellant was
originally based on chlorofluorocarbons (CFCs). CFCs are chlorine-based chemicals
which were developed in the early 1930s and used in various manufacturing processes,
such as coolants for refrigerators and solvents for cleaning electronic components.
They were also used in aerosols, including metered dose inhalers. However, in the
early 1970s it was realized that chlorine had a damaging effect on the ozone layer,
and in 1985, the Antarctic ozone hole was discovered. This led to a call to stop the
production of CFC-containing appliances.

In 1985, a general agreement was reached outlining governments' obligations to
develop systems for protecting the environment. As a result of this, the Montreal
Protocol was signed in 1987 by over one hundred countries, which began the phasing
out of the production of CFCs, and other substances that damage the ozone layer.
The aim was to achieve this by 1996. Drug companies, however, were granted an
exemption from this deadline because of the difficulties they were experiencing
in producing an effective alternative in their metered dose inhalers. This has been
particularly problematic for inhaled steroids due to differences in lung deposition
with the new propellants.

New inhalers are becoming more widely available with hydrofluorocarbons as the
propellant, but as yet, not all formulations of drug are available in this non-CFC
format. It is important, therefore, to keep abreast of developments in this area. Once

Table 6.3. Drugs available in the Easi-Breathe device

Inhaled steroids	B2 Agonists	Nonsteroidal preventer
Beclometasone	Salbutamol	Sodium cromoglycate

Inhalation technique for using an Autohaler • Shake the canister • Remove protective mouthpiece • Push the lever up and breathe out • Put the mouthpiece in the mouth, making sure there is a good seal around the mouthpiece • Take a long deep breath in (do not stop breathing in when the inhaler clicks) • Hold the breath for about ten seconds • Press the lever back down and wait sixty seconds before taking another dose • Repeat above steps for next and subsequent doses	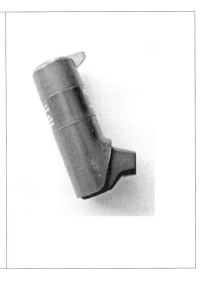

Figure 6.4. Technique for using an Autohaler device.

adequate alternative devices are available, CFC inhalers will be removed from the market completely. Recently, beclometasone has become available in two CFC-free formulations: QVAR, which has been available for some time, but is now available in a CFC-free format, and the new inhaled steroid Clenil Modulite. As mentioned earlier on in this chapter, this will probably mean the discontinuation of some forms of beclometasone. When changing patients over to any new formulation, it is important

Inhalation technique for using an Easi-Breathe device • Shake the canister • Flip protective cap off mouthpiece • Breathe out • Put the mouthpiece in the mouth, making sure there is a good seal around the mouthpiece • Take a long deep breath in • Hold the breath for about ten seconds • Replace protective cap over mouthpiece and wait for sixty seconds before taking next dose • Repeat above steps for next and subsequent doses	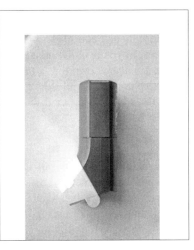

Figure 6.5. Technique for using an Easi-Breathe device.

to check the dose and licensing arrangements of the drug, as some of the newer drugs and devices are not licensed for children and the dosing regime may be different.

Patients should be informed that the new CFC-free inhalers taste and feel quite different from their previous inhalers. This may be a worry to some people who feel that they are not getting the same dose of drug into their lungs. It is important, therefore, to reassure patients that the drug itself has not changed and it is only the propellant that is different. Asthma UK, the British asthma charity, has produced a fact file about the transition, which patients may find helpful and reassuring [2].

SPACER DEVICES

Many of the problems associated with metered dose inhaler technique can be overcome with the use of a spacer device. This is a kind of holding reservoir which 'holds' the drug for a short period of time, thereby avoiding the problems in coordinating actuation and inspiration. Most spacers have a one-way valve which opens on inspiration and closes on expiration, thus allowing tidal breathing through the spacer. This is particularly useful for the very young and also elderly people who find it difficult to hold their breath following inhalation. The use of spacers has also been shown to improve lung deposition of the drug. If you remember from the section on metered dose inhalers, only about 10 % of the drug actually reaches the lungs, and this is increased to about 20 % when using a spacer device [3].

Spacer devices are recommended when using inhaled steroids at a dose of 800 mcg daily or more, via a metered dose inhaler. They help to reduce the risk of side effects from inhaled steroids because the larger, faster particles of drug stick to the walls of the spacer and are not deposited in the mouth. This also allows the fine particle dose of the drug to reach further into the lungs.

When deciding on a device for children under five years of age, there is little or no evidence to support one inhaler over another. However, the recommendation is that children in this age group should receive both inhaled steroids and bronchodilators via a metered dose inhaler and spacer [4, 5]. The choice of spacer depends on individual circumstances. In young children, a face mask may be added to the spacer.

Evidence has also shown that a metered dose inhaler and large volume spacer is just as effective in treating mild and moderate exacerbations of asthma as a nebulizer. In this case the dose of drug used should be titrated according to clinical response.

CHOICE OF SPACER

There are several different types of spacer available, and it is vitally important to ensure that the spacer and metered dose inhaler are compatible. Large volume spacers have been shown to have better lung deposition than small volume spacers, but as previously mentioned you must take into account your patient's level of understanding, and willingness and ability to use the device. Elderly people, for example, may find it difficult to get their hands around a large spacer because of arthritic fingers, and in this case a small volume spacer would be a better option. Similarly, parents trying to give inhaled drugs to little, wriggling children may find a small spacer easier to handle. Another advantage of a small volume spacer such as the AeroChamber is that it is suitable for any type of metered dose inhaler.

CARE OF SPACER DEVICES

Current advice is that spacers should be cleaned no more than once a month to enhance drug delivery. This is in contrast to manufacturer's recommendations of once a week. The main reason for this is that shiny, clean plastic spacers create a lot of static charge which causes the drug to stick to the inside surface of the spacer, resulting in less drug being available to be deposited in the lungs.

When cleaning the spacer, it should be washed in warm, soapy water, rinsed and allowed to dry naturally, perhaps draining on some kitchen paper. It should not be rubbed dry with a towel because this increases the static charge. Metal spacers are available which do not have the same problem, but these are not widely used in this country at present. Spacers should be changed at least once a year, but depending on frequency of use, may need replacing at six monthly intervals.

TECHNIQUE FOR USING A SPACER

There are two techniques for using a spacer, both of which are correct and deliver the necessary dose to the lungs. However, some patients may find one technique easier than the other to manage. Certainly infants and small children will need to use the tidal breathing technique as they will be unable to hold their breath. Similarly, elderly patients with COPD may find breath-holding difficult and in this case the tidal breathing technique is preferable.

Figure 6.6 describes these two techniques, and Figure 6.7 shows the two large volume spacers most commonly used in the United Kingdom. An example of a small volume spacer is shown in Figure 6.8 which is available with a mouthpiece and different size masks for infants and young children.

DRY POWDER INHALER DEVICES

Many drugs are available in a dry powder format which may suit some patients better than metered dose inhalers. The drug is sometimes mixed with an inert substance, for example lactose. These inhalers do not need any coordination to use and they also have the advantage that in most of them it is possible to count the doses used, and doses remaining. Another advantage is the fact that they are more 'environmentally friendly'. Patients should be advised of the possibility of oral thrush when using high-dose inhaled steroids in this format because of the increased oropharyngeal deposition.

Table 6.4 lists the most commonly used dry powder devices and the drugs that are available in them.

Technique for using a spacer device using tidal breathing	Technique for using a spacer device using breath holding
• Shake the inhaler, remove the cap and insert into the spacer • Put the mouthpiece in the mouth, making sure there is a good seal around the mouthpiece • Press the inhaler once and breathe in and out through the mouthpiece about 4–5 times • Remove the inhaler from the spacer and repeat the above steps for the next and subsequent doses	• Shake the inhaler, remove the cap and insert into the spacer • Put the mouthpiece in the mouth, making sure there is a good seal around the mouthpiece • Press the inhaler once and take a long deep breath in • Hold the breath for about ten seconds and breathe out slowly through the mouthpiece • Take another long deep breath in and hold the breath again for about ten seconds • Remove the inhaler from the spacer and repeat the above steps for the next and subsequent doses

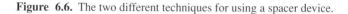

Figure 6.6. The two different techniques for using a spacer device.

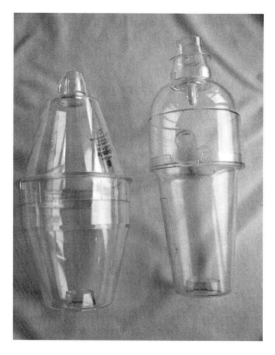

Figure 6.7. The two most commonly used large volume spacers.

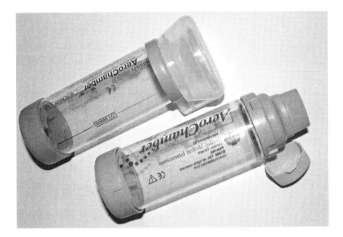

Figure 6.8. Small volume spacer showing a mask and mouthpiece.

Diskhaler

The Diskhaler is used to deliver fluticasone, beclometasone, salmeterol and salbutamol. The drug is contained within sealed foil disks with four or eight blisters, each blister containing a dose of drug. Figure 6.9 illustrates a Diskhaler and describes the technique for using it.

Accuhaler

The Accuhaler delivers fluticasone, salmeterol, salbutamol and Seretide. The drug is contained within a foil strip inside the inhaler. The device is preloaded with 60 doses, and a dose counter enables the patient to know exactly when it is empty. The Accuhaler is illustrated in Figure 6.10, together with instructions for its use.

Turbohaler

The drugs available in a Turbohaler are budesonide, terbutaline, formoterol and Symbicort. Each inhaler can contain 50–200 doses depending on the dose and the drug involved. The drug is delivered in a pure format and is completely tasteless which can be an advantage if taste is a problem. However, it can also have a disadvantage, as sometimes patients say they do not feel as if they have had a dose, and occasionally use more than the prescribed amount just to 'make sure'. A Turbohaler is illustrated in Figure 6.11, together with a description of the correct technique for using it.

Table 6.4. Most commonly used dry powder devices and the drugs available in them

	Inhaled steroids	B2 agonists	Anticholinergics	Combined	Nonsteroidal preventer
Diskhaler	Beclometasone Fluticasone	Salbutamol Salmeterol			
Accuhaler	Fluticasone	Salbutamol Salmeterol		Seretide	
Turbohaler	Budesonide	Terbutaline		Oxis Symbicort	
Handihaler			Tiotropium		
Spinhaler					Sodium cromoglycate
Clickhaler	Beclometasone	Salbutamol			
Cyclohaler	Budesonide	Salbutamol			
Twisthaler	Mometasone				

Technique for using a Diskhaler
- Remove the protective mouthpiece cover. Pull the white tray out until you can see the ridges on either side of the tray
- Squeeze the ridges together until the tray slides out completely
- Put the foil disk onto the tray with numbers uppermost, and slide the tray back into the device
- Slide the tray in and out by holding the corners. This will rotate the tray. Keep sliding it in and out until the number 8 or 4 appears in the window (depending on whether it is an eight dose device or four dose device)
- Keep the device level and lift the rear of the lid as far as it will go until it pierces the blister. Close the lid
- Breathe out, and holding the diskhaler level, put the mouthpiece in the mouth, making sure there is a good seal around the mouthpiece
- Take a long deep breath in
- Remove the mouthpiece from the mouth and hold the breath for about ten seconds
- Repeat the above steps for the next and subsequent doses

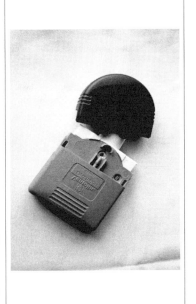

Figure 6.9. Technique for using a Diskhaler.

Technique for using an Accuhaler
- Slide back the protective mouthpiece cover
- Press lever down
- Breathe out, and keeping the device level, put the mouthpiece in the mouth, making sure there is a good seal around the mouthpiece
- Take a long deep breath in
- Remove the mouthpiece from the mouth and hold the breath for about ten seconds
- Repeat the above steps for the next and subsequent doses

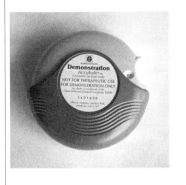

Figure 6.10. Technique for using an Accuhaler.

Technique for using a Turbohaler	
<ul><li>Hold the inhaler upright and unscrew the white cover</li><li>Twist the coloured end as far as it will go one way and then back the other way until it 'clicks'</li><li>Breathe out and put mouthpiece in the mouth</li><li>Take a long deep breath in</li><li>Remove the inhaler from the mouth and hold the breath for ten seconds</li><li>Repeat the above steps for the next and subsequent doses</li></ul>	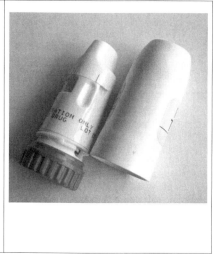

Figure 6.11. Technique for using a Turbohaler.

HandiHaler

The HandiHaler device is used for delivering tiotropium, which is mainly used in the management of COPD. However, for completeness, and because many elderly patients with asthma may have an element of COPD as well, this device has been included. The drug in this case is contained within a capsule which has to be inserted into the inhaler, where it is pierced prior to inhalation. Figure 6.12 shows a HandiHaler and describes the correct technique for its use.

Spinhaler

The Spinhaler is available for the delivery of sodium cromoglycate. With the availability of more effective drugs for the management of asthma, its use has declined; however, it is still available and some patients may be happy using it. Again the drug is contained within a capsule which has to be pierced before inhaling. A Spinhaler and its use are illustrated in Figure 6.13.

Nebulizers/Compressors

'The aim of treatment with nebulizers is to deliver a therapeutic dose of the drug as an aerosol in the form of respirable particles within a fairly short period of time, usually 5–10 min' [6].

Two types of nebulizer are available, a jet nebulizer and an ultrasonic nebulizer. The jet nebulizer is the most commonly used, mainly because it is a lot cheaper. It is a machine which drives air through narrow tubing into a nebulizer chamber which

Technique for using a HandiHaler
- Hold the inhaler upright and flip off protective cover and mouthpiece
- Insert capsule into the device
- Close the mouthpiece
- Hold the inhaler upright and press in the green button on the side
- Breathe out and put mouthpiece into the mouth
- Take a long deep breath in
- Remove mouthpiece from the mouth and hold the breath for ten seconds
- Repeat the last three steps once more to ensure complete emptying of the capsule
- Open the mouthpiece and dispose of the used capsule
- Replace protective cover

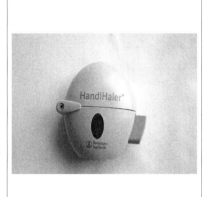

Figure 6.12. Technique for using a HandiHaler.

contains a solution of drug such as salbutamol or ipratropium. Oxygen can also be used as the driving gas, and is most commonly used in an acute asthma attack. About 12 % of the drug is actually deposited in the lungs, the rest being wasted into the surrounding air, or staying in the nebulizing apparatus. The force of the jet of air, or oxygen, breaks up the drug into a fine mist which can be inhaled and it can be quite

Technique for using a Spinhaler
- Hold the inhaler upright and unscrew the two halves
- Insert the coloured end of the capsule into the cup of the propeller
- Screw the two halves of the inhaler back together
- Move the grey sleeve up and down twice to pierce the capsule
- Breathe out and put the mouthpiece into the mouth
- Take a long deep breath in
- Remove the mouthpiece from the mouth and hold the breath for ten seconds
- Repeat the above for the next and subsequent doses

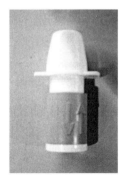

Figure 6.13. Technique for using a Spinhaler.

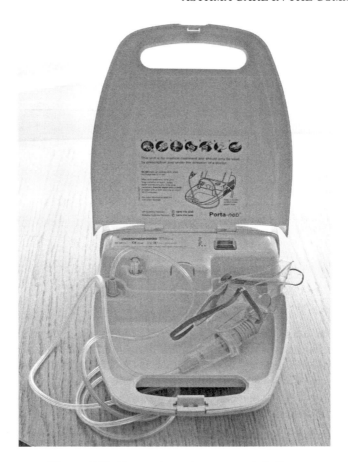

Figure 6.14. Commonly used compressor/nebulizer.

noisy in operation. Although the machine itself is commonly called a nebulizer, the nebulizer component is actually only the small chamber into which the drug is put. The correct term for the machine is a compressor. A typical jet nebulizer is shown in Figure 6.14.

The ultrasonic nebulizer works by passing high frequency sound vibrations through the drug solution, breaking it down into microscopic particles which can be inhaled. It is a lot quieter than the jet nebulizer, but is much more expensive to buy.

The other equipment that is needed to nebulize drugs consists of a mask or mouth-piece, a nebulizer chamber and a length of tubing. A mouthpiece is recommended if the patient is using ipratropium in the nebulizer because of potential damage to the eyes from the mist which escapes from the sides of the mask.

Clinical Use

Nebulizers are a convenient way of administering high-dose inhaled drugs to the lungs and are mostly used in the management of an acute asthma attack, although patients with COPD may use them on a daily basis for routine maintenance treatment. Other uses include the administration of antimicrobial drugs in cystic fibrosis, symptomatic relief in palliative care and treatment for HIV/AIDS.

When used in an acute asthma attack the driving gas should be oxygen, given at a flow rate of 6–8 l per minute. A lower flow rate produces larger aerosol particles which are too big to reach the smaller airways, and also leads to a longer nebulizing time. Domiciliary oxygen cylinders should not be used as the driving gas for nebulizers as their flow rate is not sufficient to break up the solution into the particle size that is necessary for inhalation.

Because nebulizers are such an effective and easy way of giving medication in an acute asthma attack, patients often think they should have a nebulizer at home. This is generally not recommended because there is the danger that the patient, or carers, may not seek medical help in an acute attack. The current thinking is that if a patient's asthma is bad enough to need nebulized therapy, they should seek medical help.

Another point to think about when using nebulized therapy is that it is a very expensive method of delivering drugs, when it has been shown that a metered dose inhaler and spacer is just as effective in the day-to-day management of asthma.

CARE OF A NEBULIZER/COMPRESSOR

Nebulizers should be serviced in line with the manufacturer's recommendations. This is usually once a year. Some hospitals and primary care trusts provide a nebulizer service, which includes the loan and servicing of nebulizers. The disposables should also be changed as recommended by the manufacturer. These include the mask or mouthpiece, tubing and nebulizer chambers. The less durable items may need to be changed every three months or so, but longer-lasting items are available and can last up to a year.

The nebulizer chamber should be washed and dried after every use to prevent crystallization of the drugs in the chamber, which can block the jets. Similarly, the mask or mouthpiece should be washed and dried thoroughly after every use to prevent infections. The tubing should be left dry. If there is any moisture in the tubing, it should be discarded. One way of helping to avoid this is to keep the machine running at the end of nebulizing to drive dry air through the tubing.

SUMMARY

The choice of inhaler device is probably one of the most important issues surrounding the management of the patient with asthma, and this chapter has discussed the issues surrounding the most commonly used devices. Remember, though, that other types of devices do exist, so it is important to keep an open mind and if one particular device does not seem to be suitable, search for an alternative. All it often needs is a little patience and perseverance to get this aspect of care right.

When making a decision about the best type of inhaler device for your patient, perhaps the most important message is 'The best inhaler device is the one that your patient can and will use.'

REFERENCES

1. British Thoracic Society. National Respiratory Training Centre (2005) The use of placebo inhaler devices, peak flow meters and inspiratory flow meters in clinical practice. Practical recommendations. www.brit-thoracic.org.uk/ProfessionalUpdates.
2. Asthma UK (2006) Factfile CFC-free inhalers, London. www.asthma.org.uk.
3. Newman, S.P., Miller, A.G., Leannard-Jones, T.R. *et al.* (1984) Improvement of pressurized aerosol deposition with Nebuhaler spacer device. *Thorax*, **39**, 035–941.
4. British Thoracic Society/Scottish Intercollegiate Guidelines Network (2005) *British Guideline on the Management of Asthma*, Revised edition. Available at www.brit-thoracic.org.uk/guidelines.html.
5. National Institute for Clinical Excellence (2000) Guidance on the use of inhaler systems (devices) in children under the age of 5 years with chronic asthma, NICE, London. www.nice.org.uk.
6. British Thoracic Society (1997) Nebuliser treatment best practice guidelines. *Thorax*, **52** (Supplement 2).

7   The Management of Asthma

Key points:

- Many patients with asthma tolerate high levels of morbidity.
- It is important to develop a trusting partnership between the patient and all members of the healthcare team.
- The British Thoracic Society Guideline advocates a stepwise approach to the management of asthma.
- It is important to start treatment at the step most appropriate to the severity of the disease.
- Treatment should be aimed at controlling symptoms with the lowest dose of drug possible.
- Inhaler technique and concordance with medication should be checked before moving up to the next step.
- The asthmatic patient should be reviewed regularly and medication titrated to the severity of the asthma.
- The nonpharmacological management of asthma includes primary prophylaxis and secondary prophylaxis.
- The only primary prophylactic interventions currently recommended are to encourage breastfeeding and to avoid smoking during pregnancy and in the postnatal period.
- Secondary prophylaxis includes allergen avoidance and environmental control, but there is very little evidence to support this.
- Self-management has been shown to be highly effective in controlling symptoms and reducing hospital admissions.
- Education of the patient with asthma should be consistent and given in a format the patient can understand.

INTRODUCTION

The aim of asthma management is the 'control of symptoms, including nocturnal symptoms and exercise-induced asthma, prevention of exacerbations and the achievement of best possible pulmonary function, with minimal side effects' [1].

WHAT IS CONTROL?

If the aim of asthma management is to control symptoms and achieve the best possible lung function, the question has to be asked, 'What is control?' As health professionals, we probably define control by the severity of symptoms and perhaps the number of exacerbations had by the patient. Peak flow measurements are also an important control measure. However, many patients with asthma will put up with a night-time cough, or accept that they are unable to do certain things because they consider it is normal with their condition. You quite often hear them say things like:

Of course I can't play sport, I've got asthma.

A recent survey in the United States of over 60 000 asthma patients found that approximately 68 % of paediatric patients and 78 % of adult patients reported limited activities due to asthma in the last week [2]. The survey also found that although 94 % said they would like to live symptom-free, 90 % of them expected to have symptoms. Similar surveys done by the British Asthma Charity, Asthma UK [3], have found that over 50 % of patients with asthma have more than one asthma attack every week, and 44 % find that their social life is affected by their asthma.

IS CONTROL POSSIBLE?

The next question that we may like to ask ourselves is 'Is perfect control possible?' Most guidelines say that it is in the majority of patients. However, we have to accept as health professionals that criteria for adequate control depends on personal aims and expectations, and also to balance these against the potential side effects, or inconvenience of taking medications on a regular basis to achieve 'perfect' control.

WHAT ARE THE BENEFITS OF CONTROL?

Perhaps another question we need to ask is 'Are there any benefits to long-term control?' As far as the patient is concerned, the main benefit is to be able to live a normal life, free from symptoms, and have no exacerbations. Although these are extremely important, as clinicians, we need to be thinking further than this. By making sure our patients are on optimum therapy right from the start, we can hopefully prevent the more long-term damage that results from airway wall remodelling, and possible progression to irreversible airways disease.

BRITISH THORACIC SOCIETY ASTHMA GUIDELINE

The British Thoracic Society (BTS) introduced a stepwise approach to managing asthma in 1993, which revolutionized asthma management. This method of managing asthma classifies severity of the disease, and guides the pharmacological management for each category of severity. Since 1993, the Guideline [1] has been updated several times, the latest of which was in November 2005. Other guidelines such as the Global

Initiative for Asthma (GINA) [4] also advocates a stepwise approach; however, there are slight differences in the two guidelines. For the purposes of this book the intention is to follow the BTS Guideline.

Following a diagnosis of asthma, the patient, or parent if the patient is a child, will probably go through a range of emotions. For some, it will be a relief to receive a diagnosis and treatment after perhaps weeks, or even months of being unwell. To others, it may come as a shock to be told they have a chronic disease for which they will need to take daily medication. Other patients will be totally disbelieving, saying there must be a mistake, and demand to be referred for a specialist opinion.

It is important at this stage to be patient, answer questions and try to allay any fears or worries the patient may have. After giving a simple explanation of the condition, and its management, you will need to establish what the patient's needs and expectations of treatment are. It may be useful to set goals, such as being able to sleep all night or doing some favourite hobby. It is important, however, to make sure these goals are realistic and achievable. There is nothing more demoralizing for the patient than setting a goal which they are never able to achieve. Developing a trusting partnership at this point will be invaluable in future consultations and will help lead to better control and less symptoms. Sometimes, however, trying to explain everything all at once will be just too much for the patient to take in, and you may have to arrange another follow-up appointment.

The next stage is to decide what treatment strategy you are going to employ. The likelihood is that the patient will need some sort of medication to control their asthma so the next section discusses the pharmacological management of asthma. Figure 7.1 describes what typically happens when a patient is first diagnosed with asthma and is a follow on from Figure 4.8 in Chapter 4.

PHARMACOLOGICAL MANAGEMENT OF ASTHMA

Most patients with asthma will be using some sort of medication to control their disease. This section addresses the pharmacological management of asthma, based on the BTS Guideline [1]. Steps 1–5 guide the practitioner through a sequential approach to the management of asthma. This does not mean, however, that you have to start at step 1 and then go up the steps individually until control is achieved. It is important to start treatment at the step most appropriate to the severity of the condition and then to review at frequent intervals and titrate the dose until symptoms are under control at the lowest dose of drug possible.

Step 1: Mild Intermittent Asthma

The majority of patients with asthma will be using inhalers of one sort or another. Those patients with very infrequent symptoms may only need a short-acting bronchodilator for occasional use. The current advice is that if a patient is using two or more canisters of B2 agonists a month, their asthma is poorly controlled, and they should move up to the next step.

Amy's story (part two)

In Chapter 4, I described how Amy, who is ten years old, had been diagnosed with asthma following several months of a night-time cough, and problems with exercise. Amy's peak flow rate had increased by 29% following inhalation of a bronchodilator, which showed that she had asthma.

It was decided at this stage to start Amy on an inhaled steroid and short-acting bronchodilator. Amy's mum, however, became very worried when she heard the word steroid mentioned, as she had heard it many times in relation to athletes and bodybuilders. She was also concerned that Amy wouldn't grow properly, and put on a lot of weight. It was explained to her that the type of steroids that bodybuilders and athletes sometimes used were different to the inhaled steroids used for the treatment of asthma. She seemed reassured by this and was also relieved to hear that the dose of steroid in an inhaler is very small, with little systemic absorption, compared to taking the drug orally.

Amy and her mum were given a basic description of the disease itself, and its management, and encouraged to ask questions. A discussion then followed on the type of inhaler Amy would use. The nurse showed Amy the different sorts of inhalers that were available, and demonstrated how they were used. It was eventually decided to use a metered dose inhaler and large volume spacer for her inhaled steroid, and a dry powder device for the reliever. Although a large volume spacer is perhaps not very portable, Amy didn't mind using it for her preventer because she could use it at home, and would not have to take it to school. The dry powder device, however, fitted into her pocket, or bag, and was therefore less conspicuous. Amy was also given a prescription for a peak flow meter, and a diary, and asked to record her peak flows twice daily to assess how she was responding to the treatment.

At a follow-up appointment four weeks later, Amy was much better, and Mum said that she was sleeping well, with only an occasional night-time cough. Amy's exercise tolerance had also improved, and she was now able to keep up with her friends when playing with them, or when riding their bikes. Her peak flow diary still showed some variability in her peak flow rate, but over the last week this had begun to settle, and there was less variation in her morning and evening peak flows.

The nurse spent some time with Amy and her mum, giving more information about the disease, and explaining the importance of taking her medication regularly. She also checked Amy's inhaler technique, and explained what to do if Amy's symptoms got worse. Amy and her mum were then given some information leaflets about asthma and given an appointment for three months' time to review her condition. She was also asked to try to keep a peak flow diary during this time.

Figure 7.1. Amy's story (part 2).

Step 2: Introduction of Regular Preventer Therapy

Inhaled steroids are the most effective way of controlling asthma symptoms in adults and children. However, there is very little evidence to establish the exact threshold at which inhaled steroids should be started. It is currently recommended that patients should start inhaled steroids if any of the following occur:

- exacerbations of asthma in the last two years;
- using inhaled B2 agonists three times a week or more;
- getting symptoms three times a week or more, or waking one night a week.

Inhaled steroids are generally more effective when given twice a day, but there is some evidence that with the newer, more potent inhaled steroids, once-daily dosing may be as effective. The main problem with once-daily dosing is that if a patient forgets their inhaler frequently, they may go two or three days between doses, with subsequent loss of control. There is no advantage in giving inhaled steroids more than twice a day.

Step 3: Add-on Therapy

The main option for add-on therapy at step 3 of the Guideline is a long-acting B2 agonist (LABA). This has been shown to have a greater effect at controlling symptoms than increasing the dose of the inhaled steroid. The two LABAs in current use are salmeterol and formoterol. There have been several concerns about the safety of long-acting B2 agonists recently, and several studies have implicated them in asthma deaths (see Chapter 5), but the current advice is that the benefits far outweigh any risks and that if patients have any concerns, they should discuss them with their doctor.

In light of these recent concerns, however, the Medicines and Healthcare products Regulation Agency (MHRA) [5] have issued the following recommendations:

Long-acting B2 agonists (formoterol and salmeterol) should:

- be added only if regular use of standard-dose inhaled corticosteroids has failed to control asthma adequately;
- not be initiated in patients with rapidly deteriorating asthma;
- be introduced at a low dose and the effect properly monitored before considering dose increase;
- be discontinued in the absence of benefit;
- be reviewed as clinically appropriate: stepping down therapy should be considered when good long-term asthma control has been achieved.

These recommendations are only emphasizing what has been happening in good clinical practice for some time, and if the clinician has been following evidence-based guidelines there is not likely to be any major change to the way in which these drugs are used.

Note: Salmeterol is only licensed for use in children aged four years and over, and formoterol for children aged six years and over.

Other options at this step include leukotriene receptor antagonists, slow-release theophylline or possibly, slow-release B2 agonist tablets. The choice of drug at this step will depend on several factors including the age of the patient, and what the particular problems are. Leukotriene receptor antagonist drugs, for example, may be useful in those patients who experience exercise-induced asthma, or who have an allergic component to their asthma. It does not work for everybody, however, so if there is no improvement after 4–6 weeks, the drug should be stopped.

The use of theophylline seems to come in and out of fashion, but it is a useful drug in some situations, although it should only be considered if control is not being achieved using inhaled medications. Theophyllines do have some unpleasant side effects including headaches, nausea and vomiting. These problems can occasionally be overcome by starting the patient on a low dose and building up to the recommended dosage slowly. The patient should also have regular blood tests to ensure theophylline blood levels are maintained within the therapeutic window.

It may take a bit of experimenting with different combinations of therapy, bearing in mind that some of these drugs are not licensed for use in children. It is important therefore to check the data sheet for each drug if you consider using them.

Step 4: Persistent Poor Control

In the small percentage of patients whose asthma is not well controlled at step 3, there is very little evidence as to what treatment to use, or at what dose. The BTS Guideline [1] at this stage advises increasing the dose of inhaled steroids to a maximum of 2000 mcg/day of beclometasone (or equivalent) in adults, and 800 mcg/day of beclometasone (or equivalent) in children aged 5–12 years. Children under the age of five years who are at step 4 of the Guideline should be referred to a respiratory paediatrician.

Step 5: Continuous or Frequent Use of Oral Steroids

Some patients with severe, uncontrolled asthma will need to use a small maintenance dose of oral steroid, either every day or alternate days to try to reduce the risk of side effects. These patients will need frequent monitoring, partly because of their uncontrolled asthma but also because of the potential side effects from oral steroids.

Patients at this step of the Guideline will most likely be under the care of a specialist respiratory physician. This is certainly true with children who should always be referred to a respiratory paediatrician.

A summary of the BTS stepwise approach is shown in Figures 7.2–7.4

CHOICE OF INHALED STEROID

The Guideline summarized above is based on beclometasone, but the actual choice of drug will depend on many factors, such as patient preference, and availability of drug in the most suitable inhaler device. There may be local formularies in your area of practice and you may have to abide by these. The currently available inhaled steroids are:

- Beclometasone
- Budesonide
- Fluticasone
- Mometasone
- Ciclesonide

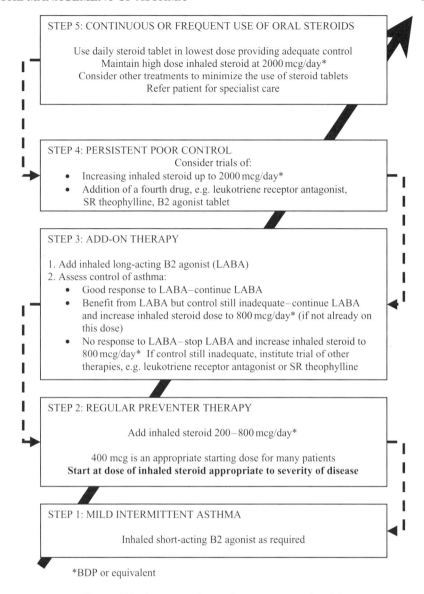

Figure 7.2. Summary of stepwise management in adults.

The two most commonly used inhaled steroids, beclometasone and budesonide are equivalent at the same dose. Fluticasone is roughly twice as potent, so therefore would be given at half the dosage of the other two. QVAR, a form of beclometasone, is also equivalent to beclometasone at half the dose. Mometasone is a fairly new drug and available evidence suggests that it should be used at half the equivalent dose of

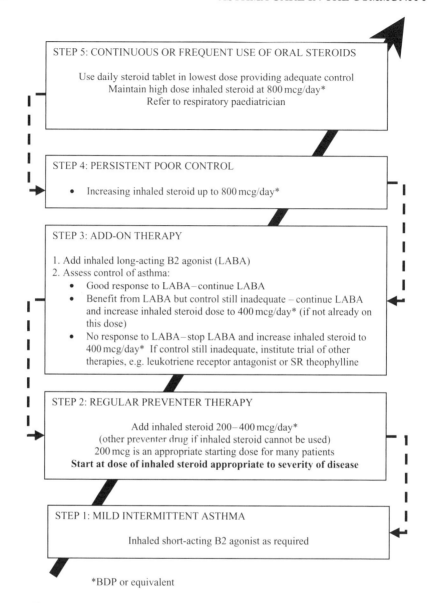

Figure 7.3. Summary of stepwise management in children aged 5–12 years.

beclometasone. Ciclesonide is also a new inhaled steroid and its efficacy and safety have not yet been established, although emerging evidence compares it to twice the dose of beclometasone.

When deciding on which to use, the main criteria should be availability of drug in a device which the patient can and will use.

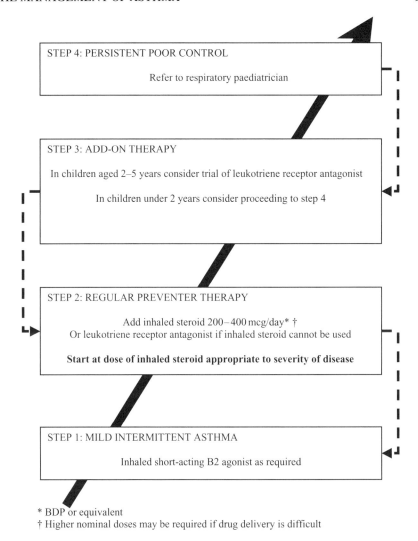

Figure 7.4. Summary of stepwise management in children less than five years.

DOSE OF INHALED STEROID

The current recommendation is to use the lowest dose of drug possible to achieve control. Often in the past, high doses of inhaled steroids were used initially to achieve control quickly, and then titrated down once control was achieved. There are advantages to this method, especially if you suspect that a patient is sceptical of the treatment, or there is a need to achieve control quickly. If it is going to take 3–4 weeks for the patient to feel any benefit, there is a risk that they will give up after a couple of weeks, thinking the treatment is not working.

The BTS Guideline [1] and GINA [4], however, recommend starting at a dose appropriate to the severity of the disease. A reasonable starting dose would be 400 mcg/day in adults and 200 mcg/day in children. In children under the age of five years, where consistent drug delivery may be difficult, higher doses may be required. At these doses, there is little risk of systemic side effects; however, as with all drugs, it is important to keep the dose as low as possible without compromising control. The side effects of steroid therapy are discussed fully in Chapter 5, but the main worries are adrenal suppression and thinning of the bones and skin. A recent study investigating the association between adrenal suppression and dose of inhaled corticosteroids in children found that those children receiving above licence doses of fluticasone were more likely to have adrenal insufficiency [6]. In children there is also the concern that growth might be affected. If control is a problem at step 2 of the Guideline, it may be more beneficial to go up to step 3 and add in a long-acting B2 agonist, rather than increasing the dose of inhaled steroid.

Most patients will be controlled at step 3, and you, as a nurse will probably be well able to manage the patient up to this stage. If, however, you need to consider moving up to step 4, it may be beneficial to refer the patient for more expert advice and help with management.

When using this stepwise approach to management, there are two important things to remember:

- Check inhaler technique and concordance with therapy before moving up to the next step: Correcting poor inhaler technique, or changing to a more suitable device may make all the difference to asthma control, and avoid having to increase doses of medication. It is also important to find out if the patient has been taking their drug therapy as prescribed. If concordance with treatment is a problem, you will need to discuss this with the patient, and if possible try to ascertain why they have not been taking their medication regularly. The remedy may be easy, such as tips on how to remember to take their inhalers, or changing to a device that will be more acceptable. There may, however, be more complex reasons for nonconcordance such as denial or other psychological issues. These problems will be much more difficult to deal with and need a lot of time and patience to overcome. The subject of nonconcordance with treatment is discussed in more detail in Chapter 8.
- Steps go down as well as up: Continual monitoring is necessary to ensure the patient is on the dose of drug most appropriate to the severity of their disease. You may be able to reduce the dose of drug during the summer months, for example, or the patient's asthma may improve and they may not need as much medication.

NONPHARMACOLOGICAL MANAGEMENT OF ASTHMA

The first part of this chapter described the management of the patient with asthma, using the traditional, pharmacological approach. Is there anything else we, as clinicians, can do for our patients that does not involve drugs? Evidence is still emerging as to the effectiveness of nonpharmacological methods of controlling asthma, such as allergen avoidance and dietary control. We shall discuss these and other methods in this section of the book; however, the role of complementary or alternative medicines are discussed in Chapter 10.

The prevention of asthma symptoms through nonpharmacological methods can be conveniently divided into two types:

- primary prophylaxis: interventions made before there is any evidence of disease;
- secondary prophylaxis: interventions made after the onset of disease to reduce its impact.

Going back to the section in Chapter 3 about the causes and triggers of asthma, you may remember we differentiated between the two by saying that the causes relate to how and why an individual develops asthma, and the triggers are the influences that make asthma worse. Primary prophylaxis therefore is associated with the former, trying to prevent asthma before it happens, and secondary prophylaxis is associated with the latter, trying to prevent asthma symptoms by avoiding the known triggers of asthma.

PRIMARY PROPHYLAXIS

There have been many theories put forward about the effectiveness of the primary prophylaxis of asthma, but as yet no convincing studies have been published to be able to recommend this type of treatment. The areas that have been investigated include environmental control and allergen avoidance, dietary modifications and the effects of early exposure to microbes. However, none of these studies has produced conclusive results.

There is some evidence that breastfeeding protects against the development of asthma [7]. This protective effect was greatest in children with a strong family history of atopy. Smoking in pregnancy, and in the postnatal period has been found to increase the risks of having a wheezy baby [8].

The only interventions that are currently recommended therefore for primary prophylaxis of asthma are to encourage breastfeeding, and to avoid smoking during pregnancy and during the postnatal period.

SECONDARY PROPHYLAXIS

Allergen Avoidance

The majority of people with asthma are atopic. Atopy refers to an immunoglobulin E (IgE) mediated sensitivity to common inhaled allergens. If you remember from Chapter 3, IgE is an important factor in the inflammatory process associated with asthma. As clinicians, we almost always advise our patients to avoid allergens where possible; however, there is surprisingly very little evidence to substantiate the effectiveness of this approach. Some studies have shown that allergen avoidance results in a reduction in disease severity [9, 10]. However, the reliability of these studies is questionable, added to which they were done at high altitude where levels of house dust mite in particular are low. Obviously it is not practical or realistic for all families with asthmatic children to live on a high mountain!

House Dust Mite

House dust mites love warm, moist atmospheres and feed on flakes of human skin. They are present in all our homes and live mainly in mattresses, pillows and soft furnishings. Normally they do not cause a problem but occasionally in susceptible people they can be a cause for concern. In actual fact it is not the mite itself which causes the problem but its faeces and they are one of the biggest triggers of childhood asthma. Babies and children naturally love cuddly toys which can be home to large numbers of house dust mites. Quite often you wonder if there is room in the cot or bed for the child, with the number of teddies and other soft toys that surround them.

There is a lot of confusion about the efficacy of house dust mite control and what effect this has on asthma symptoms. Some studies have shown that reducing exposure to house dust mites leads to less asthma symptoms. However, the measures taken to achieve this are so stringent and severe, and have such an impact on family life, that many people would rather live with their symptoms. Other studies have shown no difference in asthma symptoms. In the absence of reliable, well-conducted research, it is difficult to know how to advise patients in this matter; however, it is generally recommended to try to reduce levels of house dust mites in the home.

Patients will often tell you they have seen various advertisements for chemical sprays or machines that claim to get rid of house dust mites. These can be quite expensive and there is no evidence that any of these measures work. The most effective way of reducing the levels of house dust mite is to keep soft furnishings to a minimum, perhaps replacing carpets and rugs with wooden, tiled or vinyl floors. With children, try to limit the numbers of soft, cuddly toys to one or two favourites. If possible, try to ensure that these toys are washable, as machine washing at a high temperature will kill the house dust mite. The same applies to bedding. House dust mites are also eradicated by freezing, and putting soft toys in a plastic bag in the freezer will also help. Just remember to defrost them before putting them back in the bed! When children have to share a bedroom, perhaps using bunk beds, it is important that the child with asthma sleeps on the top bunk. Mattress covers will also help, but make sure that they cover the mattress completely.

It is important to vacuum carpets, mattresses, chairs and sofas regularly, and to use a damp duster on solid surfaces. It is best to avoid sprays and polishes as these have been known to trigger an asthma attack in susceptible people.

Pets

Pets, particularly cats and dogs, are potent triggers for asthma symptoms and airborne allergen levels increase by approximately fivefold when the pet is in the room. The most effective way of reducing pet allergen exposure is to remove the pet from the home; however, as we all know, this is not so easy. The problem with pet allergen can be very difficult to deal with and requires great sensitivity. Even when proven to be sensitive to animals, many patients will refuse to remove their pets from their homes. The problem is further compounded because following permanent removal of a pet from the home, it can still take many months for allergen levels to fall.

If the patient is adamant that they will not remove the pet from the home, they should be advised to try to keep the pet out of the bedrooms and preferably outdoors. Washing cats and dogs has also been shown to reduce allergen levels, but this effect is very short lived, so the pet would need to be washed at least once a week.

Conversely, there is some thought that those individuals who have a high, maintained exposure to pet allergens actually become desensitized.

Smoking

As previously stated, mothers who smoke during pregnancy are more likely to have a wheezy baby, and infants of mothers who smoke are four times more likely to develop wheezing illness in the first year of life [11, 12]. These studies, and many others, have shown that smoking during pregnancy has an adverse effect on lung development, and lung function in the foetus.

There is also some evidence that continued exposure to smoking during infancy contributes to the severity of childhood asthma [13]. It is therefore important to advise parents not to smoke in front of their children and also more importantly not to smoke during pregnancy. Of course, everyone should be encouraged not to smoke, whether they have asthma or not, but in the patient with asthma and in pregnancy it should be avoided at all costs. If the patient is still smoking, support and advice should be given as appropriate.

Environmental Air Pollution

There is much in the media about environmental air pollution and the adverse effect it has on our health. Pollution levels have been put forward as one of the reasons for the increase in asthma prevalence; however, there is very little evidence to substantiate this theory. The general thought is that air pollution may aggravate asthma, but much more research is needed on this subject before any firm recommendations can be made.

Diet

The role of dietary control in asthma is still not very clear, and food allergies associated with asthma attacks are relatively uncommon. In rare instances dairy products, shellfish and nuts have been known to trigger an asthma attack. This should not, however, be confused with an anaphylactic response to these foods.

Some work has been done studying the relationship between brittle asthma and food intolerance. Trying to identify which foods could be a possible trigger is very difficult, however, and this usually needs to be done in a hospital setting, in conjunction with a dietician who has a special interest in this aspect of asthma control.

It has been thought for some time that antioxidants and dietary fats have some effect on inflammation. One recent study found that at sufficiently high intakes polyunsaturated fatty acids, as found in oily fish and fish oils, reduce the inflammation associated with allergic diseases [14]. Their role in asthma, however, has yet to be proven, and a Cochrane review [15] has concluded that there is little evidence to support the use of fish oil supplements for asthma. Similarly, antioxidant supplements such as vitamin C cannot yet be recommended as the evidence for their efficacy is not available.

Allergy Tests

Quite often patients, particularly parents of asthmatic children, will ask if they can be tested for allergies. More often than not, patients will know what they are sensitive to and what triggers their asthma. However, for various reasons, they may want it confirmed by an allergy test. Conversely, some patients will not believe that a certain trigger is making their asthma worse. Therefore you may want to do an allergy test to try to convince them that perhaps they ought either to remove the trigger if it is possible, or try to avoid coming into contact with it.

The two allergy tests that are most widely used are skin prick testing and a radioallergosorbent test (RAST). Skin prick testing is the least expensive of the two and gives results within fifteen minutes. In this test a small amount of allergen is introduced into the dermis of the inner forearm. If the patient is sensitive to the substance, it will cross link to IgE molecules on the surface of cutaneous mast cells, resulting in the release of histamine. If you remember from Chapter 3, people with asthma tend to produce large amounts of IgE in response to contact with common allergens, leading to a cascade of events resulting in airway narrowing.

The test can detect sensitivity to the main allergens such as house dust mite, pollens, grass, Aspergillus, feathers, cats and dogs. Following administration of the allergen, the test site is then observed for any redness, swelling or weal. The size of the weal is measured and if it is 3 mm or larger, it is regarded as a positive result. Positive and negative controls are also included in the test to ensure reliability. It is important to ensure that the patient has not taken any medications such as antihistamines prior to the test which may interfere with the result.

The other test to measure atopy is the RAST. This is a blood test, where a sample of blood is taken and exposed to different allergens. The test is able to detect sensitivity to the most common allergens as in the skin prick test described previously. If the patient is sensitive to the substance, levels of IgE will rise.

Immunotherapy

Immunotherapy has been available for many years, but because of the risks associated with the procedure, is not used to any great extent. It involves injecting gradually increasing quantities of an allergen extract, which modifies the immune response. Although this intervention has been shown to be effective in some cases, there remains a high risk of anaphylaxis and death. If it is done at all, it will be performed in specialist centres and by clinicians who have a lot of experience in this treatment.

Patient Education and Self-Management

In today's modern Health Service, everybody is being encouraged to be more proactive in their own healthcare, and the population in general are now far more aware of health matters, and also what they have a right to expect from their healthcare providers. The majority of patients now expect to be told about their condition, and how it is treated. In certain conditions, especially chronic diseases, patients are also being encouraged to take responsibility for their own care. This has been reflected in the Department of Health's [16] recent publication on supporting people with long-term conditions, where self-management is promoted as being central to improving quality of life and maintaining independence.

Self-management in asthma is not new, and many studies have shown it to be beneficial in reducing morbidity, hospital admissions and acute exacerbations. A recent review, for example, found that asthma self-management results in a reduction in acute exacerbations and admissions, less time off work, and an improvement in quality of life [17]. Despite this, many patients are never given advice on self-management, as shown by a survey conducted by Asthma UK [3]. So, how do we implement asthma self-management, and what are the problems that might make it fail?

The first point to recognize is that perhaps the wording 'self-management' may be a problem in itself. Some patients may find this a little daunting, preferring their asthma to be managed by someone else, preferably a doctor or nurse. In view of this, the title now more commonly used is 'Asthma Action Plan'. The emphasis in this case is more on giving the patient a plan to follow, with actions to be taken in the event of worsening symptoms.

The starting point in helping patients to manage their own condition has to be education, and this has been shown to be crucial in the success of self-management in asthma. Unless patients understand what asthma is, and what it does to their bodies, they cannot be expected to take responsibility for the management. How this education is given will depend very much on the working environment. A practice nurse, for example, may only have a ten or fifteen minute appointment in which to do everything, so time for education is limited. However, every time the patient is seen for review is an opportunity for education, and this opportunity should not be missed.

The other time when education is important, and perhaps may be more effective, is following an acute exacerbation. Before discharge from the accident and emergency department, or from the hospital ward, the patient's inhaler technique and adherence to medication should be checked as a matter of course. However, this is also a good time to reinforce the importance of being able to recognize deteriorating asthma and know what to do, before it gets bad enough to need emergency treatment.

It is important that any education given should be consistent and structured. It should also be given in a format that the patient can understand and relate to. A simple description of the disease itself, and what they can expect from their treatment, should then be accompanied by a written action plan. The form this plan takes will depend on the individual patient, and their level of understanding and commitment. At the very least it should explain the signs and symptoms that would indicate worsening asthma and give advice on what actions to take. A more detailed action plan may include a diary of symptoms and peak flow recordings, with clear directions on what to do if the peak flow falls below a certain level. Some patients will be happy to record their peak flow regularly, but this may not be so acceptable to others.

In the past, patients were often told to double up their dose of inhaled steroid at the start of a cold, or if their peak flow rate was falling. The evidence for doing this was however scant, and the most recent evidence has shown that in patients who are taking a regular dose of inhaled steroid, doubling the dose has no effect [18, 19]. However, another review [20] of 26 randomized controlled trials found that increasing the dose of inhaled steroid in some instances was effective, and the British Thoracic Society [1] does state in their Guideline that it may be acceptable to include this option in an action plan. This is confusing to say the least, but it is important to be aware that this is an issue that needs further research. If you do decide to incorporate it into an action plan, you need to be certain of your reasons for doing so.

You may wish to use a template action plan and adapt it for each patient. Asthma UK, the British asthma charity, have produced an excellent range of materials to help both health professionals and patients in managing asthma. An example of their Asthma Action Plan is shown in Figure 7.5. However, the most successful asthma action plans are those which are personal and tailored to the individual patient. You may therefore wish to design or create a plan yourself, which has been discussed and agreed with the patient, thus building up a partnership in which the patient actually becomes an active participant in the healthcare team.

ASTHMA ACTION PLANS AND CHILDREN

An asthma action plan for children can be very similar to one that is used for adults and contains the same information and advice. However, the plan may need to be adapted to suit different age groups. For example, parents will have responsibility for asthma management in younger children, but as the child grows up they may want to have more of a say in their own asthma management. The education package will also need to be aimed towards a more family-centred approach, but always remembering that the child must be involved in all discussions when they are of an age to do so. This is particularly true with teenagers, who should be given responsibility for looking after their own asthma, with an action plan developed to suit the individual patient.

When developing an action plan for children under the age of five years, it is not possible to base it on their peak flow rate as peak flows in children of this age are unreliable and not generally advised. The plan therefore needs to be based on symptoms alone, with advice on actions to be taken at certain stages of worsening

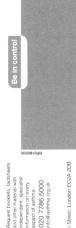

Figure 7.5. Asthma UK Action plan.

Zone 1

Your asthma is under control if:

- You have no or minimal symptoms during the day or night (wheezing,coughing, shortness of breath, tightness in the chest)
- You can do all of your normal activities without asthma symptoms
- Your peak flow reading is above [ ] (85% of your best)

Action

Continue to take your usual asthma medicines.

Preventer medicine should be used every day,even when you are feeling well.Your preventer medicine is

name [ ]
colour [ ] Take [number of puffs/doses]
dosage [ ] [when]

Reliever medicine should be used if you have symptoms. Your reliever medicine is

name [ ]
colour [ ] Take [number of puffs/doses]
when [ ]

Other medicines taken regularly may be added to your treatment if your preventer is not stopping all of your symptoms.Your add-on medicine is [name]

colour [ ] Take [number of puffs/doses]
when [ ]

If you are always in zone 1,your doctor or nurse may want to reduce (step down) your regular medicines.

Zone 2

Your asthma gets worse if:

- You need to use your reliever inhaler more than once a day
- You have had difficulty sleeping because of your asthma
- Your peak flow reading is between [ ] and [ ] (between 70% and 85% of your best)

Action

Increase your preventer inhaler

name [ ]
colour [ ] Take [number of puffs/doses]
dosage [ ] [when]

Stay on this dose until you have had no symptoms for [days] then return to your dose in zone 1.

Continue to take your reliever medicine

name [ ]
colour [ ] when needed.

If your symptoms do not improve in [days] contact your doctor or nurse for advice.

Your doctor or nurse will discuss your inhaler with you and check your inhaler technique. You may be started on a different medicine to help you get your symptoms back under control.

If you are often in zone 2,let your doctor or nurse know at your next review.Your usual medicines may need to be increased or changed.

Zone 3

Your asthma is much more severe if:

- You need to take your reliever inhaler every four hours or more often
- You have symptoms all the time
- Your peak flow reading is between [ ] and [ ] (between 50% and 70% of your best)

Action

Continue taking your preventer medicine as prescribed at the higher dose in zone 2.

Continue to take your reliever medicine when needed.

If you have been prescribed steroid tablets,take [number] 5mg prednisolone tablets immediately and again every morning for [days] or until your symptoms have improved or your peak flow has been at [ ] for two days.

Your doctor or nurse may want you to let them know within 24-36 hours that you have started a course of steroid tablets.If you regularly take steroid tablets,your doctor or nurse will advise you on how to reduce the number you are taking.

If you are often in zone 3,let your doctor or nurse know.Your usual medicines may need to be increased or changed.

Zone 4

It is an asthma emergency if any of the following happen

1 Your reliever (blue) inhaler does not help
2 Your symptoms get worse (cough, breathless, wheeze, tight chest)
3 You are too breathless to speak
4 Your peak flow reading is below [ ]

Action

1 Take your reliever (blue) inhaler
2 Sit up and loosen tight clothing
3 If no immediate improvement during an attack,continue to take one puff/dose of reliever inhaler every minute for five minutes or until symptoms improve
4 If your symptoms do not improve in five minutes – or if you are in doubt – call 999 or a doctor urgently

Your asthma medicines - what to use on an everyday basis

	Your medicine is:	How much to use:	When to use:	Comments/symptoms:
Preventer				
Reliever				
Other				

How to recognise if your asthma is getting worse

Have you had difficulty sleeping because of your asthma symptoms (including coughing)?
Have you had your usual asthma symptoms during the day (wheezing, coughing, shortness of breath, tightness in the chest)?
Has your asthma interfered with your usual activities (eg housework, work or school)?
If 'yes' to one or more of the above, or if you have not seen your doctor or nurse about your asthma for 12 months or more,arrange to have a review.If 'yes' to all of the above – is this an emergency? (see overleaf)

Figure 7.5. *(Continued)*

symptoms. The easiest way to do this is to ask the parents to keep a symptom diary, which scores levels of symptoms. An example of a symptom diary is shown in Chapter 4.

SUMMARY

The introduction, in the early 1990s, of guidelines for the management of asthma has revolutionized the way we manage this common, chronic disease. Using a stepwise system makes the process much simpler and enables a consistent approach among the different healthcare professionals who may come into contact with the asthmatic patient. In particular this approach has also made it possible for nurses to be more autonomous in their practice, and able to manage the asthmatic patient on their own, within the boundaries of protocols, and their own knowledge and expertise.

We have also discussed the nonpharmacological approach to managing asthma, and the message at this particular time seems to be that there is still a lot of work to be done to prove whether or not this aspect of asthma management is effective.

Lastly we looked at education and self-management for patients with asthma. There is no doubt that this works, but what is still lacking is evidence on what constitutes a good action plan and what sort of information needs to be included.

REFERENCES

1. British Thoracic Society/Scottish Intercollegiate Guidelines Network (2005) *British Guideline on the Management of Asthma*, Revised edition. Available at www.brit-thoracic.org.uk/guidelines.html.
2. Carlton, B.G., Lucas, D.O., Ellis, E.F. *et al.* (2005) The status of asthma control and asthma prescribing practices in the United States: results of a large prospective asthma control survey of primary care practices. *Journal of Asthma*, **42** (7), 529–35.
3. Asthma UK (2004) *Living on a Knife Edge*, London. www.asthma.org.uk.
4. Global Initiative for Asthma (2006) *Global Strategy for Asthma Management and Prevention*, Revised edition. www.ginaasthma.org.
5. Medicines and Healthcare products Regulation Agency (2006) Asthma: Long-acting B2 agonists. www.mhra.gov.uk.
6. Paton, J., Jardine, E., McNeill, E. *et al.* (2006) Adrenal responses to low dose synthetic ACTH (Synacthen) in children receiving high dose inhaled fluticasone. *Archives of Disease in Childhood*, **91**, 808–13.
7. Gdalevich, M., Mimouni, D., Mimouni, M. (2001) Breast-feeding and the risk of bronchial asthma in childhood: a systematic review with meta-analysis of prospective studies. *Journal of Pediatrics*, **139** (2), 261–6.
8. Gilliland, F.D., Berhane, K., McConnell, R. *et al.* (2000) Maternal smoking during pregnancy, environmental tobacco smoke exposure and childhood lung function. *Thorax*, **55** (4), 271–6.

9. Peroni, D.G., Boner, A.L., Vallone, G. *et al.* (1994) Effective allergen avoidance at high altitude reduces allergen-induced bronchial hyperresponsiveness. *American Journal of Critical Care Medicine*, **149** (6), 1442–6.

10. Simon, H.U., Grotzer, M., Nikolaizik, W.H. *et al.* (1994) High altitude climate therapy reduces peripheral blood T lymphocyte activation, eosinophelia, and bronchial obstruction in children with house dust mite allergic asthma. *Pediatric Pulmonology*, **17** (5), 304–11.

11. Stocks, J., Dezateux, C. (2003) The effect of parental smoking on lung function and development during infancy. *Respirology*, **8** (3), 266–85.

12. Dezateux, C., Stocks, J., Wade, A.M. *et al.* (2001) Airway function at one year: association with premorbid airway function, wheezing, and maternal smoking. *Thorax*, **56** (9), 680–6.

13. Cook, D.G. and Strachan, D.P. (1999) Health effects of passive smoking – 10: Summary of the effects of parental smoking on the respiratory health of children and implications for research. *Thorax*, **54** (4), 357–66.

14. Calder, P.C. (2006) n − 3 polyunsaturated fatty acids, inflammation and inflammatory diseases. *American Journal of Clinical Nutrition*, **83** (6 suppl), 1505s–19s.

15. Woods, R.K., Thien, F.C., Abramson, M.J. (2002) Dietary marine fatty acids (fish oil) for asthma in adults and children. *Cochrane Database Review*, **2002** (3), CD001283.

16. Department of Health (2005) *Supporting People with Long Term Conditions*, London.

17. Gibson, P.G., Coughlan, J., Wilson, A.J. *et al.* (2003) Self-management education and regular practitioner review for adults with asthma. *Cochrane Database Review*, **2003** (1), CD001117.

18. Harrison, T.W., Oborne, J., Newton, S., Tatersfield, A.E. (2004) Doubling the dose of inhaled corticosteroid to prevent asthma exacerbations: randomised controlled trial. *Lancet*, **363**, 271–5.

19. Fitzgerald, J.M., Becker, A., Sears, M.R. *et al.* (2004) Canadian asthma exacerbation study group. Doubling the dose of budesonide versus maintenance treatment in asthma exacerbations. *Thorax*, **59** (7), 550–6.

20. Gibson, P.G., Powell, H. (2004) Written action plans for asthma: an evidence based review of the key components. *Thorax*, **59**, 4–99.

8 Special Situations

Key points:

- Asthma is the most common chronic disease to affect children.
- There are many different causes of wheeze in children.
- Children should be reviewed more often than adults to ensure normal growth and development.
- Teenagers are a distinct group of patients with different requirements from adult or paediatric patients.
- In the elderly, it is important to ensure that the right diagnosis is made.
- Drug therapy in the elderly may be more complex because of the likelihood of polypharmacy.
- Elderly patients often find inhalers difficult to use correctly.
- The phases of the menstrual cycle can affect asthma symptoms in some women.
- It is important to maintain control of asthma during pregnancy to avoid the risks of foetal and maternal complications.
- Inhaled drug therapy in pregnancy is safe, as are oral corticosteroids, but care should be taken with other oral preparations.
- Occupational asthma is the most common industrial lung disease in the world.
- Brittle asthma can affect 0.05 % of all asthmatic patients and is very challenging to manage.
- Asthma is a physiological condition of the lungs; however, psychological influences can impact on asthma control.
- Concordance with treatment is important to maintain control.

INTRODUCTION

The management of asthma is generally straightforward; however, there are some situations that are more difficult to manage and which require a different, more individual approach – for example, the care of children and the elderly. This chapter addresses some of the more common 'difficult to manage' issues surrounding asthma management in a number of situations that may require a different management strategy in order to gain control of symptoms.

ASTHMA IN CHILDREN

Wheezing episodes in children are very common, especially in the under-twos. In this age group there are many different causes of wheeze and it is important to be able to distinguish the wheeze of asthma from other causes of wheeze. In the majority of cases the wheeze will be viral in origin and the child will usually recover quickly with no serious consequences. However, in the first year of life, children may become infected with respiratory syncytial virus (RSV) which can make them very ill indeed, and they may need hospital admission.

Cough is also a problem in young children, and like wheeze, many children will cough with viral infections. This cough may carry on well after the infection has cleared up. How, therefore, do we tell the difference between viral wheeze and cough, and asthma? This section of the book addresses this issue but if there is any doubt at all, the child should be referred to a paediatrician for clarification of the diagnosis.

Risk Factors

Asthma is the most common chronic disease to affect children. It is also the most common diagnosis of children admitted to hospital.

Although we still do not know exactly why some children develop asthma and others do not, there are some risk factors that are known to increase the risk of developing asthma in childhood. A family history of asthma is an important indicator, with the risk more strongly associated with maternal asthma and atopy. Babies who are born prematurely are more likely to develop asthma or wheeze. Breastfeeding, however, has been shown to protect babies and infants from developing asthma.

Boys are much more likely to develop asthma in infancy and are more likely to grow out of it in their early teens. Girls, however, have a greater risk of persisting asthma through childhood to adulthood. The reasons for this are unclear but it is thought to relate to the fact that at birth the airway diameter of boys is smaller than girls, leading to increased susceptibility to airway hyperreactivity. This difference evens out during puberty and then the airway diameter in boys eventually overtakes that of girls, leading to more symptoms of asthma in the female sex.

Maternal smoking during pregnancy leads to an increased risk of the infant developing asthma and/or wheezing type illnesses. It has also been shown to increase asthma severity during the early years. In addition to this, asthmatic children who live in a smoking household are more likely to have problematic asthma leading to hospital admissions.

DIAGNOSIS OF ASTHMA IN CHILDREN

Physicians are often reluctant to diagnose asthma in children under the age of two. This is because recurrent wheeze is very common and only in the minority of cases becomes asthma. In fact the earlier the symptoms appear in infancy, the better the

Table 8.1. Indications for referral for specialist opinion

Indications for referral for specialist opinion
- Any doubt about diagnosis
- Symptoms presenting from birth
- Severe upper respiratory tract infection
- Family history of unusual chest disease
- Failure to thrive
- Excessive vomiting
- Persistent cough, especially if productive
- Clinical signs and symptoms do not correspond to the history
- No response to conventional treatment
- Frequent use of oral corticosteroids
- Parental anxiety

prognosis. Most children who wheeze in infancy become asymptomatic by the age of five years. In contrast, the more severe asthma is in childhood, particularly in the 3–5 year age range, the more likely it is that it will continue into adulthood.

Diagnosis in childhood is based more on a clinical history and symptoms, rather than on objective measurements of lung function. The clinician should be alert to a possible diagnosis of asthma in the case of the child who presents with a night-time cough, cough and breathlessness on exercise, and worsening symptoms with colds. It is important to take a detailed history, always remembering that there are other possible causes of cough and wheeze in children. Clinical examination, including chest auscultation, should be performed, but may not always be helpful in diagnosing asthma because of the variability of the condition. A child who has been coughing all night, for example, may present the following morning with no symptoms whatsoever.

Peak flow measurements in the under fives are not usually very reliable and not normally recorded. It is also important not to confuse a young child by asking him/her to blow into one device, for example a peak flow meter, and then suck in on another device, an inhaler. Diagnosis is usually confirmed by a trial of treatment and a symptom diary may be helpful. An example of a symptom diary is given in Chapter 4, Table 4.2.

Do not forget, however, that symptoms of asthma can be similar to other childhood diseases such as cystic fibrosis, immunodeficiency, primary ciliary dyskinesia and aspiration. If there is any doubt, or if the child is failing to respond to drug therapy, referral should be made to a consultant paediatrician who has experience in looking after children with respiratory disorders. Table 8.1 lists the indications for referral for specialist opinion.

PHARMACOLOGICAL MANAGEMENT OF CHILDREN WITH ASTHMA

Although the basic management of asthma is the same in adults and children, there are certain aspects that need special consideration. As with adults, the management of asthma is aimed at controlling symptoms, using the lowest dose of drug possible to achieve the desired effect. Total daily doses of inhaled steroids should not exceed 800 mcgs of beclometasone or equivalent for children aged 5–15 years. In children under five, the dose should not exceed 400 mcgs of beclometasone or equivalent. As doses of more than 400 mcgs a day have been associated with systemic side effects, it is recommended that other add-on therapies such as long-acting B2 agonists should be considered before increasing the dose of inhaled steroids.

Occasionally parents will say that they do not want their child to be taking steroids in any form. This can be quite a difficult issue to address, as there is no doubt that inhaled steroids are the treatment of choice to control symptoms, prevent exacerbations and avoid the long-term lung damage that can occur in uncontrolled asthma. There should be an open and frank discussion about the role of steroids in asthma, and the parents reassured as much as possible about the relative safety of inhaled steroids in particular. However, if after discussion, they are still adamant that they do not want their child on inhaled steroids, there is the option of using sodium cromoglycate, which is a nonsteroidal inhaler. There are disadvantages of using this drug, namely having to take it at least three to four times a day for it to be effective, and it will take up to six weeks to show any beneficial results. It also has the added problem of having a nasty taste which children often find unpleasant.

Figures 7.3 and 7.4 in Chapter 7 show the BTS stepwise approach to managing asthma in children.

Inhaler Devices

Even in small babies, the inhaled route is the preferred method of drug delivery. This allows for much lower doses to be used with subsequent less risk of side effects, which is particularly important in childhood. Inhaler devices in general are discussed in detail in Chapter 6; however, for children under the age of five, a spacer and metered dose inhaler are the best options for administering asthma medications. There are a wide range of spacer devices available, large and small, with or without masks, which make it relatively easy to administer drugs to even the tiniest baby. The choice of spacer device depends on the drug chosen, and ability and preference of the parent or guardian. Although large volume spacers have been shown to provide greater lung deposition, they can be difficult to manage when trying to hold a wriggling, fighting infant.

When deciding on an inhaler device for a child, try to ensure that they have some input into the discussion where they are of an age to do so. Although effectiveness of the chosen drug and device is of course important, sometimes there has to be a bit of give and take where children are concerned. To them, the colour, taste and look of an inhaler are far more important than what it does. The inhalers their friends use will also matter to them, so a bit of compromising may be necessary to make sure they are happy with their inhaler.

The National Institute for Clinical Excellence (NICE) has produced guidelines [1] for inhalers in the under-fives which is summarized in Table 8.2. The device of choice

Table 8.2. Recommended inhaler devices for children under five (NICE, 2000)

Age group	1st choice	2nd choice	3rd choice	Breath-actuated	Dry powder
0–2 years inclusive	MDI + spacer + face mask	MDI + spacer	Nebulizer (rarely needed)	Avoid	Avoid
3–5 years inclusive	MDI + spacer	MDI + spacer + face mask	Nebulizer (rarely needed)	Not proven	Possible use for B2 agonists but not recommended for corticosteroids

for younger children is a spacer with metered dose inhaler. As children get older, they may well be able to manage one of the smaller dry powder devices, especially in school where they may feel self-conscious about using large volume spacers.

Parents should be advised to try to make using an inhaler fun. Using techniques such as counting, or singing nursery rhymes, help to make the child more relaxed and not dread having to take their inhaler. Having relaxed parents will also help the situation. Babies and children are very quick to sense when parents are tense or anxious, so being positive and smiling when inhaler time comes will help. Praise and encouragement are also important to children. Sometimes putting stickers onto spacers is useful as it makes the devices more personal and not so clinical.

Inhaler Technique

Inhaler technique should be checked at every opportunity. Children by nature are always in a rush to get on to the next thing, especially when it comes to medicines. Because of this, inhaler technique may suffer.

NONPHARMACOLOGICAL MANAGEMENT OF CHILDREN WITH ASTHMA

Allergen Avoidance

There is some evidence that reducing house dust mite levels in the home leads to decreased symptoms of asthma in childhood. However, it is important to be realistic and practical when advising parents about house dust mite control. Keeping soft furnishings to a minimum and regular vacuuming of carpets, sofas and mattresses are tasks that are fairly easy to achieve. Damp dusting is also feasible. Mattress and pillow covers may help but these items can be expensive to buy. Expecting families to live in a dust-free, hygienic 'bubble', however, is neither practical, realistic nor reasonable. In fact it has been shown that reducing house dust mite exposure in childhood actually makes no difference at all to symptoms of cough and wheeze [2].

Pets

Children naturally love animals but unfortunately they are a known trigger for asthma. Parents often feel guilty at having to deny their child a pet of their own, but sometimes this has to be the best course of action. On the other hand, children sometimes appear to be unaffected by their own family pet which has lived with them since infancy, but are unable to tolerate their friends' or relatives' pets. It has even been suggested that introducing exposure to dog or cat allergens in early life results in increasing immunity to animals.

Children and pets is always an emotive subject and it is sometimes difficult to know what to advise. If the family does not have a pet, it may be best to advise them not to get one. If they already have a much loved dog or cat, however, it is unreasonable to expect them to get rid of it. You may have to settle with advising them to try to restrict it to one or two rooms and definitely to keep it out of bedrooms.

Diet

Occasionally parents worry that something their child is eating may be contributing to their asthma symptoms. Generally speaking, food allergens rarely cause an increase in asthma symptoms, but it does sometimes happen. The types of foods that most commonly affect asthma are dairy products, shellfish and nuts. Food additives have also been known to trigger asthma. If a parent is concerned and thinks that diet does have a part to play in their child's asthma, it is important to refer them to a dietician so that they do not exclude vital nutrients which are essential for normal growth and development.

Exercise

Children normally have loads of energy and always want to be on the 'go'. There is the temptation with some parents to restrict their child's activities because it might trigger their asthma. Although this is understandable because obviously a parent will always want to protect their child, they must be reassured that energetic activity will not necessarily make asthma worse. There may be some activities which will have to be restricted such as doing a cross-country run on a cold day, for example, but on the whole exercise should be encouraged. Swimming especially is an excellent exercise for children with asthma, but care should be taken as some children will be allergic to the chlorine in swimming pools.

Some sports, however, are easier for the asthmatic child to cope with than others. Sports that require short bursts of energy, for example, may have to be recommended rather than endurance type sports. Children who do have problems with exercise-induced asthma should be advised to take their reliever inhaler 15–30 min before starting the activity. This can sometimes be problematic in school, as the child may feel embarrassed about using their inhaler in front of their classmates, and it has been known for school staff themselves to be reluctant for children to have access to their inhalers during school time. Involving the school nurse or health visitor may help to overcome this problem.

Monitoring

It is important that children with asthma are reviewed regularly, possibly every six months, but certainly at least once a year. Structured review and monitoring are discussed more fully in Chapter 11, but there are special considerations when reviewing children. Inhaler technique and concordance with medication should be assessed as a matter of course, and if the child or parents have been keeping a peak flow or symptom diary, they should be asked to bring it with them.

For children to develop normally and achieve their full potential in whatever path of life they choose to take, it is important that they keep as healthy as possible. When you are looking after children with asthma, this becomes a very important issue in their management. The child who is waking frequently at night cannot perform efficiently during the day, and school work and other activities will be adversely affected. Children who need to take a lot of time off from school miss out not only on the academic side of things, but also lose friendships and become socially disadvantaged.

Family life in general can also suffer when a child has asthma. Other family members may be kept awake by the child coughing at night and outings or special occasions may have to be cancelled at short notice because of the child's asthma. This can have a harmful effect on siblings who may feel jealous, or sidelined because of the attention that the asthmatic child is getting.

When reviewing the child with asthma, therefore, it is important to ask the right questions. Questions like 'Are you sleeping alright?' or 'What is your exercise tolerance like?' will only produce limited responses. You will get a much better idea of what is happening by asking more specific questions such as:

- How many times a night do you wake up because of your asthma?
- How many nights a week do you wake up because of your asthma?
- How often do you have to stop before your friends do when playing/riding your bike/running around?
- How many times a day, or week, do you need to use your reliever inhaler?

This sort of direct questioning will get a more direct response from the patient, or parents, and therefore give you much more of an idea of how well the child's asthma is being controlled.

It is important to monitor children's height, especially if they are using high doses of inhaled steroids. It is also important to be on the lookout for signs of adrenal suppression, including drowsiness and fatigue.

Asthma Action Plans and Education

When considering an asthma action plan for children, it is important to take into account levels of understanding of both the child and the parents. If the child is of an age to understand, then try to develop a plan that is aimed at the child, perhaps using graphics or colour coding to emphasize different points. As with adults, the plan should be individualized to suit each patient, but also should reflect the family's coping abilities.

Asthma and Teenagers

The teenage years can be problematic for all sorts of reasons. Fluctuations in hormone levels may cause mood swings, and the previously well-behaved, polite child becomes obstinate, rebellious and rude, generally making family life a misery. The stress of examinations and having to decide on future careers causes a lot of anxiety. During this time, body image and peer pressure is very important and teenagers do not want to be seen as different. Media pressure plays a big part in their lives and they are constantly bombarded with information about the latest fashions, accessories and gadgets. Add to this a chronic disease like asthma and it all sometimes becomes a bit too much. Some teenagers cope very well, but unfortunately some find it a bridge too far and use all sorts of behavioural strategies to manage their condition.

One of the biggest problems is with concordance with medication. Inhaled therapy has been demonstrated to be preferable to oral therapy in asthma, but unfortunately this means using devices which are not easy to conceal. Body image and self-esteem are perceived by teenagers as being extremely important and necessary for their psychological and social well-being. They do not like being or looking different from their peer group and so may not want to be seen using inhalers when with their friends. Psychological influences also have a big part to play in teenage asthma and patients may use denial techniques so that they do not feel different from their peers.

The teenage years are naturally associated with risk-taking behaviour and some of these risks may be fairly minor, for example not coming home at the right time or missing lessons. Occasionally, however, the risks may be of a more serious nature such as smoking or experimenting with alcohol or illicit drugs. These topics are not easy to address but an attempt should be made to try to guide the teenager to more acceptable, less risky behaviour with regard to their health. It is important, therefore, to be able to talk on their level, using language they can understand and relate to.

Try to involve the teenager in any discussions about their healthcare, and if possible discover how they feel about having asthma and what they expect from their treatment. Negotiate treatment plans with them and ensure that the inhaler devices they are prescribed are suitable and acceptable to them. There may need to be a compromise on both sides – for example, letting them have an inhaler they like even though it may not be the most suitable, in return for a promise to take it regularly. Teenagers should be recognized as being a distinct group of patients with different requirements from adult and paediatric patients and you may have to find novel ways of dealing with them.

ASTHMA AND THE ELDERLY

The main problem in this age group is getting the diagnosis right. When an elderly person presents with symptoms of cough, wheeze or breathlessness, asthma is probably the last thing that the clinician will think of. Asthma can develop at any age, so it is important always to consider this as a diagnosis. Other possible diagnoses include heart failure, anaemia, chronic obstructive pulmonary disease (COPD), lung cancer or fibrosing conditions like pulmonary fibrosis.

If you suspect asthma, or have eliminated other possible causes of the symptoms, you obviously need to make a diagnosis. The diagnostic process in the elderly is the same as in other age groups, so you may decide to do a reversibility test as described in Chapter 4. However, complete reversibility may not always be possible, especially if the patient is or has been a smoker. Sometimes the patient may have asthma with an element of COPD, or even COPD with an element of asthma, and there will possibly be more reversibility with an anticholinergic drug such as ipratropium bromide. Another consideration is to check the patient's current drug treatment, as patients in this age group are often taking a number of drugs for conditions such as hypertension or heart failure. Some of these drugs may have side effects which may confuse the situation. For example, one of the side effects of Angiotensin Converting Enzyme (ACE) inhibitors used for hypertension and heart failure is a cough, so it is important to be able to differentiate the reasons for or causes of the symptoms.

Once you have decided that this is definitely asthma, the next thing to consider is drug therapy. The stepwise approach in the pharmacological management of asthma is the same in this age group as for other age groups. However, there are certain issues that need to be considered. Do not forget that in the elderly, there is a lower metabolic clearance, which means that the absorption and excretion rate of drugs will differ. In the case of inhaled drugs, this is not too much of a problem; however, care should be taken with oral preparations such as theophylline and prednisolone. The latter particularly should be used with care as this can lead to reduced bone mineral content, therefore increasing the risk of osteoporosis and bone fractures. If your elderly patient needs to take frequent courses of oral corticosteroids, or if their asthma is bad enough to need a maintenance dose of prednisolone, you may wish to consider using some bone protection treatment, for example one of the bisphosphonate group of drugs.

As previously discussed, elderly people are often taking drugs for other conditions so it is important that any drug you do decide to give the patient does not interact with anything else they may be taking. Inhaled drugs are relatively safe and do not usually interact with other drugs. Theophylline, on the other hand, has many drug interactions, so care should always be taken when using this drug.

It is also important to check what other drugs the patient may be taking in relation to asthma triggers. Nonsteroidal anti-inflammatory drugs for conditions like arthritis are known to trigger asthma in susceptible people. Look out also for beta blockers, even in eyedrops, and aspirin, which are also possible triggers for asthma. You may be able to stop these drugs but sometimes, when weighing up the risks and benefits, this is not an option. You may therefore have to continue the drugs and monitor more closely.

Inhaler devices can be a big problem with elderly people. One study found that more than 50 % of elderly patients are unable to use their inhaler device properly [3]. Another study, investigating elderly people's ability to use inhalers for delivering the influenza vaccine zanamivir, found that the majority of elderly people were not able to use the inhalers [4]. In the former study, the most common errors were failing to shake the device, poor coordination of actuation and inhalation, and being unable to hold the breath. Using a spacer gets over the problem of coordination and breath holding, but some elderly people find that they are unable to cope with a large volume spacer because of arthritic hands. A small volume spacer may therefore be advisable, or a dry powder device may be more suitable for some patients. Whatever the chosen device, it is important that the patient is taught how to use it and is able to demonstrate correct technique. It is also important to check inhaler technique at every review and to be prepared to change the device if necessary.

When deciding on any drug regime for patients, it is always best to keep it as simple as possible. This is even more important with elderly people. If possible try to ensure that all inhaled drugs are available in the same device. You may decide that a combination inhaler may be easier for them to manage, rather than having two inhalers, for example Seretide, Symbicort or Combivent.

ASTHMA AND WOMEN

During childhood, boys show a higher prevalence of asthma with an incidence of two boys to one girl. During adolescence, the incidence equalizes and then becomes more common in females. A recent study conducted in Norway found that in the age groups 13–16 years, current wheeze was reported in 29 % of girls and 20 % of boys [5]. Several reasons have been suggested for this changeover in prevalence. It has been suggested that boys have a higher level of bronchial responsiveness during infancy and childhood which diminishes at puberty. It is also thought that hormonal influences may have a part to play in the increased susceptibility, that is apparent in girls during and after puberty.

Acute exacerbations of asthma are a common cause of admission to hospital, and it has been shown that women of reproductive age are admitted to hospital more often than men [6]. Many studies have been conducted to investigate the cause of the higher admission rate, but there has been no really satisfactory answer as to why this happens. Most studies have concentrated on the hormonal aspect, for example comparing admissions to phases of the menstrual cycle, the menopause or pregnancy. The results of these studies have been inconsistent and have not provided any real answers.

Menstrual Asthma

It has long been recognized that some women experience worsening asthma just before and during the first few days of menstruation, although no absolute reasons have ever been identified. New evidence, however, is emerging that worsening asthma is also reported in women just prior to ovulation. This is confusing to say the least and the authors of this latest study are not able to explain this phenomenon [7]. They suggest that both the preovulatory, and perimenstrual phases act as triggers, or they may be cofactors that worsen other recognized triggers of acute asthma.

During both these phases of the menstrual cycle there is a great fluctuation in hormone levels, particularly oestrogen and progesterone, and it is generally thought that this is the cause of worsening asthma associated with the menstrual cycle. However, this has never been proved and the discussion is ongoing.

Another suggestion as to why some women experience worsening asthma symptoms in relation to their menstrual cycle is that they may be suffering from premenstrual syndrome. The symptoms of premenstrual syndrome include irritability, depression and bloating. There may therefore be heightened awareness of the physical symptoms of asthma and the perception of severity may alter. Also at this time, women are more likely to take over the counter medicines, such as aspirin and non-steroidal anti-inflammatory drugs. Both these groups of drugs are known to trigger asthma symptoms in a small group of patients.

Although it would be good to have a better understanding of asthma and the menstrual cycle, it should not detract from the way in which we manage these women. What is known is that many women do have deteriorating asthma just before and during menstruation. It is also known that many more women present to accident and emergency departments with worsening asthma related to their menstrual cycle. It is essential therefore that the needs of these women are addressed and nurses are pivotal in tackling this important issue.

Managing Menstrual Asthma

Women frequently do not relate their asthma symptoms to their menstrual cycle, so the most important aspect of dealing with premenstrual asthma is to actually find out if this really is a case of asthma associated with the menstrual cycle. You need to ask the right questions, and encourage open discussion. A diary of peak flow and symptoms may help to identify and link deteriorating asthma control to the menstrual cycle.

Various methods of treating premenstrual asthma have been tried. Prophylactic medication and the use of B2 agonists can be increased prior to menstruation and in some women this is all that is needed. A written self-management, or action plan, is key to this sort of management. Do not forget also to check inhaler technique and concordance with medication at every opportunity.

However, there is a subset of women in whom the increase of traditional asthma medication makes no difference at all. In fact there does not appear to be a consistent approach and none of the studies that have been done has provided any valid answers. Some of the treatment strategies that have been tried are intramuscular progesterone or oestrogen, ovarian secretion suppressors, and an oral contraceptive. Unfortunately as yet there is no satisfactory, consistent method of managing the severe asthma symptoms that are occasionally associated with the menstrual cycle. Research is ongoing and hopefully will provide some answers in the near future.

Asthma in Pregnancy

During pregnancy, it is not uncommon for the severity of asthma to change. For some women it will get better, for others it will get worse. There does not appear to be any way of predicting what effect asthma will have on pregnancy, or what effect pregnancy will have on asthma. A pregnancy during which the asthma becomes worse does not automatically mean that subsequent pregnancies will follow the same pattern. It is generally thought that about one-third of women will experience an improvement in their asthma symptoms during pregnancy, one-third will experience a worsening of their asthma symptoms and one-third will show no difference at all.

Management of Asthma during Pregnancy

It is very important to maintain asthma control during pregnancy for both the mother and the baby. Uncontrolled asthma is associated with many foetal and maternal complications such as hypertension, pre-eclampsia and intrauterine growth restriction, to name but a few. If, on the other hand, asthma is well controlled during pregnancy, there is little or no increased risk of complications.

The standard drugs such as B2 agonists and corticosteroids used to treat asthma are perfectly safe in pregnancy and outweigh the risks to the foetus from severe or uncontrolled asthma. Theophylline is recommended only for use when the patient's asthma is not controlled on the normal standard medications. The decision as to whether theophylline should be used is usually made by a specialist medical practitioner. During pregnancy, absorption rates of drugs are often altered, so the medication may need to be given at lower doses than normal. Leukotriene receptor antagonists, however, should not be commenced in pregnancy as data is limited in this area.

> It is extremely important to consult the data sheet before prescribing any drugs in pregnancy.

The implications for nursing practice in this situation are very important. When pregnant, women not only have their own health to consider, but also the health of their unborn baby. This is a situation where nurses can be very effective in helping women cope with the concerns they may have and giving full explanations of their management. It is also important that there should be good liaison between all the agencies involved in the care of the woman, for example, GP, midwife and consultant.

OCCUPATIONAL ASTHMA

Occupational asthma is asthma that is caused by the environment in which the affected person is working. It differs from conventional asthma in that the symptoms usually

Table 8.3. Occupations most commonly causing occupational asthma and occupations at increased risk of developing occupational asthma

Occupations most commonly reported to cause occupational asthma	Occupations at increased risk of developing occupational asthma
Paint sprayers	Bakers
Bakers and pastry makers	Food processors
Nurses	Forestry workers
Chemical workers	Chemical workers
Animal handlers	Plastics and rubber workers
Welders	Metal workers
Timber workers	Welders
	Textile workers
	Electrical and electronic production workers
	Storage workers
	Farm workers
	Waiters
	Cleaners
	Painters
	Dental workers
	Laboratory technicians

disappear when the person is removed from the triggers or vice versa. Correct diagnosis is important because the patient may be able to claim industrial compensation.

The true prevalence of occupational asthma is not known, but is thought to be in the region of 15 % of adult onset asthma [8]. This figure is taken from epidemiological studies and compensation registries. There are over 400 reported causes and it is the most common industrial lung disease in the world. The occupations most commonly reported to cause occupational asthma, and those at increased risk of occupational asthma, are listed in Table 8.3. The most common causative agents are listed in Table 8.4.

Diagnosis of Occupational Asthma

It is extremely important to diagnose occupational asthma as early as possible as delay leads to increasing symptoms, rapid decline in lung function and a poor long-term prognosis [9]. If you, or the patient, suspects that he or she has occupational

Table 8.4. Most frequently reported causative agents for occupational asthma

The most frequently reported causative agents for occupational asthma	
Epoxy resins	Animals
Flour and grain dust	Colophony fumes
Latex	Wood dust
Isocyanates and aldehydes	

asthma, it is important to ascertain when the symptoms occur, and if they get better when not at work. However, this is not as clear-cut as it appears. For example, the patient may be symptom-free at the beginning of the working week and then get gradually increasing symptoms which carry on until Saturday when they are not working. This makes occupational asthma more difficult to diagnose. A more reliable way of assessing this is asking if the symptoms improve during a long holiday.

Probably the easiest way to confirm occupational asthma is to ask the patient to keep a peak flow diary. Typically, the peak flow rate will be low or more erratic on days when the patient is working, and higher and more stable when the patient is not working. This can be quite a time-consuming exercise, however, as it is recommended that peak flow measurements should be recorded every two hours from waking to sleeping, for four weeks. However, for the patient to claim compensation, more specific tests are sometimes performed and these are usually done in a hospital outpatient setting.

Management of Occupational Asthma

Ideally, the aim of management is to identify the cause, remove the worker from the trigger(s) and for the patient to find other suitable employment. Often, removal from the causative environment results in complete recovery, although, if the worker has been exposed to the causative agent for a long time, it is unlikely that lung function will become completely normal again. However, this is not as simple as it seems. In areas of high deprivation, and high unemployment, for example, workers may be unwilling to give up their job, and this needs to be handled with great sensitivity.

BRITTLE ASTHMA

The term 'brittle asthma' was first used by Margaret Turner-Warwick [10] in 1977 to describe a pattern of asthma characterized by wide variations in peak flow rate despite high doses of inhaled steroids. The inference was that there was a specific group of patients whose asthma was difficult to control. This was followed up by various studies indicating that patients who showed this chaotic pattern of peak flow were more likely to die from an acute severe asthma attack.

During this time it also became obvious that there was a second group of patients whose asthma deteriorated suddenly on a background of apparent normal or well-controlled asthma. Subsequently the term 'brittle asthma' was used to describe solely this group of patients, who were at risk of severe, life-threatening attacks of asthma, usually 'out of the blue'. As time has gone on, however, more studies have shown that variable peak flow rate is a risk factor for death, so now two types of brittle asthma are recognized:

- Type 1: wide PEF variability ($>40\%$ diurnal variation for $>50\%$ of the time over a period >150 days) despite intense therapy;
- Type 2: sudden severe attacks on a background of apparently well-controlled asthma.

Prevalence of Brittle Asthma

There is little information about the prevalence of brittle asthma, partly due to the problems with definition. It has been suggested that 0.05 % of all asthmatic patients suffer from brittle asthma, with females, aged 18–55 years, more likely to suffer from type 1. There does not appear to be any sex difference in type 2.

Risk Factors

Patients with type 1 brittle asthma are more likely to have high levels of atopy, and problems associated with food intolerance. These patients are also more likely to have suffered from a psychiatric or psychological disorder. No risk factors for type 2 brittle asthma have been identified.

Management of Brittle Asthma

The management of the patient with brittle asthma can be very challenging, and most of these patients will be under the care of a consultant chest physician. Because of the problems in management and extra support needed, these patients are often seen as difficult, 'heart sink' patients. They are usually on high doses of inhaled steroids and bronchodilators, have tried every possible combination and dose of pharmacological intervention and their doctor has run out of further therapeutic options.

Treatment with one of the steroid-sparing drugs as described in Chapter 10 may be effective, and some patients find that a long-term subcutaneous infusion of a B2 agonist, usually terbutaline, helps. Occasionally, patients with brittle asthma are provided with a preloaded adrenaline syringe for administration in an acute attack. This involves education of both the patient and partner/carer. When patients have complex problems, it is sometimes easy to forget the basics of asthma management. So, do not forget that inhaler technique and concordance with therapy should be checked at every review. Control of allergen exposure may help and patients should be advised to avoid known allergens if at all possible. A written, self-management or action plan should be agreed with the patient and it should be constantly reviewed and updated.

Asthma is a physiological condition of the lungs; however, psychological problems can have an impact on asthma control and management. Patients with brittle asthma often exhibit psychological and behavioural problems. They have been shown, for example, to use abnormal coping strategies, such as delaying seeking medical help when they have an acute asthma attack, or even denial of having a problem at all. These issues will be discussed in the next section of this chapter. It should be remembered, however, that not all patients with brittle asthma have psychological problems and also that psychological problems can be exhibited by patients with only mild to moderate asthma.

PSYCHOLOGICAL FACTORS AND ASTHMA

Coping with any chronic disease is difficult, and some patients appear to cope better than others. It has been suggested that the way a person adapts to living with a chronic disease depends on the underlying psychology of the individual concerned [11]. For example, some people have an inbuilt 'happy personality', and no matter what happens to them, or around them, they manage to maintain a positive outlook. On the other hand, there are those who never seem to be happy, despite having all the advantages of good health, being in a stable relationship and having a comfortable lifestyle.

The psychological effect of having asthma therefore will depend largely on the person's underlying personality. The positive person will say, 'OK, I have asthma, but I'm going to get on with my life.' The person with a more negative attitude, however, is likely to be constantly thinking about their asthma, and will allow it to take over their life to the point of avoiding possible situations where they may encounter problems. For example, they may stop doing sport, or going out with their friends in case they have an asthma attack. While this is understandable to a certain extent – after all, being acutely breathless is very distressing – it does mean that this individual has a very much poorer quality of life than the patient who just gets on with it.

There is no doubt that emotion can, and does, trigger acute asthma attacks. The nature of the emotional event can be extremely varied. It can be a frightening situation, such as being physically attacked, or it can be a stressful situation such as sitting an important examination or going for an interview for a job. For some people with asthma, the realization that they have forgotten to take their reliever inhaler out with them will trigger an asthma attack.

Patients with mental health problems are a particularly vulnerable group and have special needs which are complex and very challenging. To be able to instigate any form of effective treatment, it is important to try to find out what their beliefs are about their asthma and its treatment, and have an understanding of family dynamics and social background. It is also important to ensure that any underlying anxiety or depression is being treated effectively.

Fatal or near fatal episodes of asthma are often associated with psychiatric or psychological disorders for varying reasons which are difficult to determine. As discussed in the section on brittle asthma, patients may be in denial of their condition or perhaps delay seeking medical help when their symptoms deteriorate. This may be because they have difficulty recognizing when they need help, or there may be other factors which are much more complex. It could perhaps be attention-seeking behaviour, for example a teenager using their condition as a method of getting their own way in a particular situation, or even as a form of revenge on a partner for a perceived wrongdoing.

Depressive symptoms are a fairly common occurrence in many patients who have a chronic health condition, and people with severe, difficult to control asthma may well have undiagnosed, or unrecognized depression. It is important always to be aware of the possibility of depression in this group of patients, and to ensure that the relevant treatment is offered. This may include using antidepressants, or referral for other therapies such as counselling, psychiatric or psychological help.

CONCORDANCE WITH TREATMENT

The term concordance is favoured over the previous terms of compliance and adherence, because it is meant to convey that the management of asthma is a partnership between the patient and the health professional. Nonconcordance therefore is a failure of both parties to come to an understanding, rather than an inability of the patient to follow an action plan or treatment regime. The act of concordance, or nonconcordance, could be applied to a patient's use of drug therapy or to their behaviour, for example not seeking medical help when their asthma is getting bad.

The reasons why people do not take their prophylactic asthma medication can vary from simply forgetting to not seeing the need to take medication when they are feeling well. There is no doubt that the more complex the drug therapy, the more likelihood there is of nonconcordance. Trying to keep things as simple as possible, ensuring that the same devices are used for all drugs, and possibly using combined therapies will help get over some of the problems of nonconcordance.

The issues surrounding nonconcordance, however, are often extremely difficult to deal with. Psychological factors may play a part, for example the patient may be depressed, or not motivated to keep their asthma under control. A recent study has shown that depression is a factor in concordance with asthma medication, and plays a large part in acute exacerbations and hospital admissions [12]. Denial of asthma is another problem, and patients will sometimes, for whatever reason, refuse to accept the diagnosis. This is further compounded by the fact that they may have periods of being perfectly well between asthma attacks.

There are no easy answers. Taking time to explain to the patient how their medication works, and the importance of taking it regularly may help. Finding the right inhaler device for them is extremely important. Occasionally, having a relative or friend with them when they attend for review (with their permission of course) may help to get the message across. Sometimes whatever you try will not work and more novel ways may have to be found to help this particular group. A compromise may have to be reached, and action plans developed that reflect the individual's beliefs about their asthma and its management.

Unfortunately, people with a mental illness are more likely to be smoking, which is obviously not going to help any lung condition they may have. In a large prevalence study conducted in the United States it was found that people with mental illness were twice as likely to smoke as those without mental health problems, and also that they were more likely to be smoking much more heavily than other smokers [13]. This is a difficult issue to address and will require great skill and ingenuity. Good liaison with other members of the healthcare team, such as psychiatric nurses, will be of value when trying to sort out this problem, and indeed any other problems where mental health issues are impinging on a patient's physical health.

Another factor to consider in our multi-ethnic society is the patient's cultural and religious beliefs. During Ramadan, for example, Muslims fast between the hours of sunrise and sunset, and some Muslims decide not to use their inhalers during this time, even though the laws of Islam do allow people with long-term conditions to use their medication. This again is an issue which will need great sensitivity to address. Prophylactic medications such as inhaled steroids and long-acting bronchodilators can be taken early in the morning before sunrise and after dark at night. Sudden attacks of wheezing during daylight hours, however, will be a problem if the patient refuses to use their short-acting bronchodilators.

SUMMARY

This chapter has discussed the issues surrounding asthma management in a number of special situations including asthma in children and teenagers, asthma in the elderly, asthma and women, occupational asthma, brittle asthma and asthma and mental health. These are all areas that perhaps require a more in-depth knowledge of asthma, but perhaps more importantly need a different, more individualized approach to their management. Remember, however, that in whatever field of healthcare you are working, or in whatever context you may come into contact with these patients, there is usually someone else you can turn to for advice or support. Liaison with all other members of the healthcare team is vital to the successful management of all these groups of patients.

REFERENCES

1. National Institute for Clinical Excellence (2000) Guidance on the use of inhaler systems (devices) in children under the age of 5 years with chronic asthma, NICE, London. www.nice.org.uk.
2. Gotzsche, P.C., Johansen, H.K., Schmidt, L.M., Burr, M.L. (2004) House dust mite control measures for asthma (Cochrane Review). *The Cochrane Database of Systematic Reviews*, (Issue 4). Art.No. CD001187. DOI:10.1002/14651858. CD001187.
3. Dow, L., Fowler, L., Lamb, H. (2001) Elderly people's technique in using dry powder inhalers. *British Medical Journal*, **323**, 49.
4. Diggory, P., Fernandez, C., Humphrey, A. *et al.* (2001) Comparison of elderly people's technique in using two dry powder inhalers to deliver zanamivir: randomised controlled trial. *British Medical Journal*, **322**, 577.
5. Tollefsen, E., Bjermer, L., Langhammer, A. *et al.* (2006) Adolescent respiratory symptoms – girls are at risk: The Young-HUNT study, Norway. *Respiratory Medicine*, **100** (Iss. 3), 471–6.
6. Morrison, D.S., McLoone, P. (2001) Changing patterns of hospital admission for asthma, 1981–1997. *Thorax*, **56**, 687–90.
7. Brenner, B.E., Holmes, T.M., Mazal, B., Camargo, C.A. (2005) Relation between phase of the menstrual cycle and asthma presentations in the emergency department. *Thorax*, **60**, 806–9.
8. Newman Taylor, A.J., Nicholson, P.J., Cullinan, P. *et al.* (2004) Guidelines for the prevention, identification and management of occupational asthma: Evidence review and recommendations, British Occupational Health Research Foundation, London. www.bohrf.org.uk.

9. Anees, W., Moore, V.C., Burge, P.S. (2006) FEV1 decline in occupational asthma. *Thorax*, **61**, 751–5.
10. Turner-Warwick, M. (1977) On observing patterns of airflow obstruction in chronic asthma. *British Journal Chest Diseases*, **71**, 73–86.
11. Hyland, M.E. (1998) *Asthma Management for Practice Nurses: A Psychological Perspective*, Harcourt Brace, London. ISBN: 044305682X.
12. Smith, A., Krishnan, J.A., Bilderback, A. *et al.* (2006) Depressive symptoms and adherence to asthma therapy after hospital discharge. *Chest*, **130**, 1034–8.
13. Lasser, K., Boyd, J.W., Woolhanler, S. *et al.* (2000) Smoking and mental illness: A population-based prevalence study. *JAMA*, **284**, 2606–10.

BIBLIOGRAPHY

Ayres, J.G., Miles, F. and Barnes, P.J. (1998) Brittle asthma. *Thorax*, **53**, 315–21.

9   Deteriorating Asthma

Key points:

- Most asthma deaths follow a history of severe, chronic disease.
- Occasionally a patient who has previously had well-controlled asthma will have a near fatal, or fatal asthma attack.
- Most asthma attacks follow a period of recognizable deterioration.
- Risk factors include previous episodes of near fatal, repeated hospital admissions and those who have a poor psycho/social background.
- When managing the patient with deteriorating asthma control, always be aware of the possibility of alternative diagnoses.
- Accurate assessment of the patient with acute asthma is vital to assess the severity of the attack and to monitor response to treatment.
- Following assessment, treatment should be started immediately with high flow oxygen and high dose nebulized bronchodilators.
- Oral corticosteroids should be given as early as possible in the acute attack.
- All patients with acute severe, or life-threatening asthma should be admitted to hospital.
- Patients who have had an acute attack of asthma should be reviewed at the earliest opportunity.
- Patient education and written action plans have been shown to be an effective management strategy in preventing acute episodes and reducing hospital admissions.

INTRODUCTION

The death rate from asthma is falling, however, it is still evident that the majority of asthma deaths are avoidable for various reasons, including inadequate monitoring and follow-up, and underestimation of the fatal attack, both by the patient or carer, and also by health professionals. Many asthma deaths follow a history of chronic, severe disease, but occasionally a patient who has previously only exhibited mild or moderate symptoms, will have a near fatal, or fatal attack. It is important therefore to be able to recognize deteriorating asthma and know what to do when it occurs. This chapter addresses the issues surrounding deteriorating asthma and also describes the assessment and treatment of the patient experiencing an acute attack.

WHAT IS DETERIORATING ASTHMA?

Although sudden attacks can happen, most asthma attacks follow hours or even days of recognizable deterioration. Many patients, for example, report increasing symptoms, such as wheeze, breathlessness and coughing, especially at night or with exercise, days before the onset of an acute asthma attack. Some patients may only experience one of these symptoms and, in children particularly, a night-time cough can be the only clue. Other not so obvious signs include increasing tiredness, irritability and a general feeling of being unwell.

Objective measurements are a great help in recognizing deteriorating asthma and the easiest and cheapest method of doing this is to provide the patient with a peak flow meter. This is a very reliable form of objective asthma monitoring and most patients, with the exception of the under fives, should be able to manage to record their peak flows. Along with an increase in asthma symptoms, many patients find their peak flow starts to fall, or becomes more variable days before an asthma attack. This is illustrated in Figure 9.1.

Increasing use of a bronchodilator is another clue to deteriorating asthma, especially if the patient says it is not working, or its relieving effect does not last as long as it usually does. The signs of deteriorating asthma are listed below.

Signs of Deteriorating Asthma

- increased symptoms especially at night or with exercise;
- falling and/or wide variability in peak flow rate;
- increased use of bronchodilators;
- the relieving effect of bronchodilators does not last as long as usual.

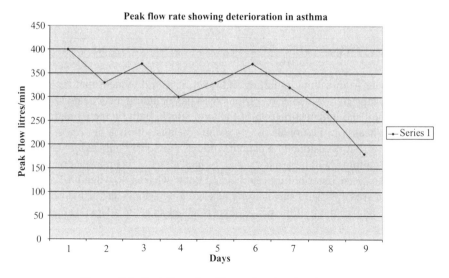

Figure 9.1. Peak flow chart illustrating deteriorating asthma.

Risk Factors

Some patients are more likely than others to suffer from deteriorating asthma control leading to an acute exacerbation. These include, for example, patients who have had repeated hospital admissions, have brittle asthma, or who have had previous near fatal attacks. Other patients known to be at risk of developing acute severe asthma include those suffering from depression or other psychiatric illnesses and those who live in poor housing conditions. The presence of any of these risk factors should alert the clinician that the patient needs more intensive monitoring and support in the management of their asthma.

The risk factors for acute, severe asthma are summarized in Table 9.1

Managing Deteriorating Asthma

When a patient presents with uncontrolled, deteriorating asthma, it is tempting to look at the BTS Stepwise approach [1] and think that it is necessary to move up a step and add in another drug or increase the dose of current medication. It is far more important, however, to step back and ask yourself a question –

What is happening to this patient, and why?

This is the time to go back to basics. The two most important points to consider in deteriorating asthma are inhaler technique and concordance with medication. These are also the easiest things to put right before going on to the more complex issues

Table 9.1. Risk factors for developing near fatal or fatal asthma

A combination of severe asthma:
- Previous near fatal asthma
- Previous admission for asthma especially in the last year
- Requiring three or more classes of asthma medication
- Heavy use of B2 agonist
- Repeated attendances at A & E for asthma care especially in the last year
- Brittle asthma

PLUS adverse behavioural or psychosocial features
- Noncompliance with treatment or monitoring
- Failure to attend appointments
- Self-discharge from hospital
- Psychosis, depression, other psychiatric illness or deliberate self-harm
- Current or recent major tranquillizer use
- Denial
- Alcohol or drug abuse
- Obesity
- Learning difficulties
- Employment problems
- Income problems
- Social isolation
- Childhood abuse
- Severe domestic, marital or legal stress

such as changing drug regimes or increasing dosage of medicines. Therefore the first thing to do is to check the patient's inhaler technique and, if there is a problem, either correct the technique or, if applicable, change the device.

The second thing to do is check if your patient has been taking their prophylactic medication as prescribed. This can be a bit more difficult as patients may not want to admit they have not been taking their inhalers regularly. One way of doing this is to say something like:

> It's very difficult to remember to take medications regularly and many people do forget. In an average week, how often would you say you forget to take yours?

This way you are giving your patient permission to admit they sometimes forget. Another way of checking concordance is to look at the patient's prescription use. Do they always pick up their prescriptions for their inhaled steroids, or do they only ask for prescriptions for their reliever inhalers? If this is the case, talking to the patient and explaining why they need to take both types of medications may help. However, there may be more deep-rooted problems that are more difficult to deal with. Is the patient steroid phobic, for example, or perhaps they may not be able to afford the cost of the prescriptions. Some people, however, do genuinely forget to take their medications and some memory prompting ideas may be necessary. For example, most people brush their teeth every night and morning, so it may be a good idea to keep their preventer inhaler with their toothbrush.

Patients often find it difficult to understand why they should take medicines when they are feeling well. They may take their prophylactic medication for a few weeks, or perhaps months, feel better and think they don't have asthma any more. They also sometimes think they only need to take asthma medication when they have symptoms. There is therefore a constant need for patient education and this should be part of every review. However, even when you feel that everything is going well with a patient, and they seem to understand the concepts of asthma management, occasionally something happens and you have to look at a more individualistic approach to addressing the problem. This is illustrated in Figure 9.2, where both the nurse and the patient have had to make a compromise. The nurse has agreed to a different method of drug delivery, and a less rigorous monitoring regime, in return for a promise of concordance with medication.

Lack of concordance and patient behaviour in chronic disease management, however, can be very complex and is often much more difficult to address. For example, there can be psychological issues, and various other problems which are discussed more fully in Chapter 8.

Another reason for deteriorating asthma could be the triggers with which the patient may have come into contact. Has the family acquired a new pet, for example, or moved house or have there been any stressful or emotional situations which could have contributed to the deterioration? Often, removal from the precipitating factor may be all that is needed to improve control. Sometimes, however, this may not be possible and other solutions may need to be found.

Amy's story (part 3)

As we learned earlier on in the book, Amy, then aged ten, had been diagnosed with asthma and had been started on an inhaled steroid and short-acting bronchodilator. Although Amy had responded well to this, at her three month follow-up appointment, it was obvious that Amy was still getting some breakthrough symptoms and was needing to use her reliever inhaler several times a week. In view of this, rather than increase the dose of inhaled steroid, the nurse decided to move up to step 3 of the BTS Guideline and add in a long-acting bronchodilator. This treatment regime appeared to work and Amy remained well and symptom-free for the next six months.

The following winter Amy's symptoms unfortunately deteriorated and she eventually needed to be admitted to hospital with an acute exacerbation of her asthma. Following discharge from hospital, Amy came to the surgery with her mum for a review of her condition and to try to find out what had gone wrong. The nurse checked Amy's inhaler technique and asked about concordance with medication. Amy admitted that she frequently did not take her preventer inhaler, mainly because she did not like the spacer. She also said she did not see why she had to take her medication on a regular basis when most of the time she was well, and complained about having to do her peak flows every day.

The nurse spent some considerable time explaining the importance of taking her preventer inhaler, and the reason for recording her peak flow measurements, but Amy was still obviouslyunhappy. She asked if she could have a different inhaler device for her preventer and long-acting reliever, as a friend had told her you could get both medications in the same inhaler, and she did not want to carry on using a spacer. An agreement was eventually reached between Amy, her mum and the nurse, and Amy was given a combined preventer and reliever dry powder device. It was also agreed that Amy would only measure her peak flow rate a couple of times a week. In return, Amy promised to take her treatment regularly.

Following these changes, Amy managed to control her asthma reasonably well, with only occasional worsening of symptoms which usually responded well to a few puffs of her short-acting reliever inhaler.

Figure 9.2. Amy's story (part 3)

Optimization of Drug Therapy

Once you have investigated and corrected all the 'easy' issues surrounding deteriorating asthma, you can move on to optimizing drug therapy. You may need to increase the dose of inhaled steroid, or add in another drug such as a long-acting B2 agonist or leukotriene receptor antagonist. If the symptoms are severe enough, the patient may need a short course of oral corticosteroids, with early review.

Patient Self-Management

Patient self-management is an important aspect of maintaining control in asthma and written self-management plans have been shown to lead to better symptom control, less exacerbations and improved quality of life. In addition, not possessing a self-management plan has been shown to lead to a greater risk of hospital admissions and acute presentations [2]. All patients with severe asthma should have a written, agreed, self-management or action plan to guide them in what to do when things start to go wrong. This should include guidance in when to increase their medication, and when to seek medical help. Management plans are discussed more fully in Chapter 8.

Differential Diagnosis

When trying to correct deteriorating control, always be aware of the possibility of other diagnoses. Failure to respond to conventional asthma treatment, especially when you are climbing the ladder of the stepwise approach, may be a sign that the diagnosis is wrong. If you are at all doubtful, refer to someone with more experience and knowledge. Possible differential diagnoses are described in Chapter 4. Figure 9.3 gives an example of a patient who was being treated for deteriorating asthma, but in fact had another, undiagnosed condition. The difficulty in this case was the fact that there were many red herrings, for example, nonconcordance with treatment, being on suboptimal therapy and smoking. The nurse followed the correct procedure by trying to correct these issues first, but the main problem was the alpha-1 antitrypsin deficiency. It is important to keep an open mind, and always be on the lookout for other causes when you come across a patient with asthma which is out of control.

The Acute Exacerbation

Many patients with asthma experience episodes when they suddenly become breath-less, wheezy or start to cough. In the majority of cases, a couple of puffs of their reliever inhaler will relieve symptoms enough to enable them to return to their nor-mal activities. Occasionally, however, patients will experience an acute attack severe enough for them to need medical help. When presented with a wheezy, breathless patient, it is very tempting to start treatment immediately without recording peak flow or any other objective measurements, because obviously you want to relieve the symptoms as quickly as possible. However, thorough assessment of these patients is very important to ensure that the right treatment is given and to be able to assess the response to the treatment.

Patient Assessment

The patient with acute asthma may present to a hospital accident and emergency department or doctor's surgery. In both cases, the basic assessment procedure should be the same. Don't forget, however, that the first person the patient may come into contact with is likely to be a receptionist, so it is important that all reception staff have guidelines or protocols to follow in the event of a patient presenting with an acute attack of asthma.

Emily's story

Emily is 15 years old and lives with her mother and younger brother. Emily's parents separated when she was two years old, and she has had verylittle contact with her father since then. Emily has had asthma since she was a baby, and control has always been erratic. However, over the last two to three years Emily's asthma has become more difficult to control, and she has needed three hospital admissions in the last six months. Following her last admission, she was referred to the community respiratory specialist nurse for assessment, and advice with management.

On assessment Emily was found to have a peak flow rate of 300 litres per minute which was 72 % of the predicted value for someone of Emily's age, height and sex. Her prescribed medication consisted of budesonide 200 mcg, 2 puffs twice a day, given via turbohaler, and salbutamol as necessary for relief of symptoms. Emily admitted that she did not take her preventer on a regular basis, mainly because she did not understand the reasons for doing so. It transpired that concordance with her medication had become much worse in her early teens when her mother had no longer felt the need to supervise Emily's asthma. On questioning, Emily also admitted that she regularly smoked at least ten cigarettes a day. Furthermore, Emily's mother smoked when in the same room as her, and had also smoked during pregnancy.

After discussion, and explanation of why she should take her medication regularly, Emily promised to adhere to an agreed management plan. She also agreed to try to stop smoking, and the relevant support was offered. It was decided that a long-acting bronchodilator should be added to the treatment regime, but because of Emily's reluctance to comply with medication, this was given in a combined formulation which delivered an inhaled steroid together with a long-acting bronchodilator in one device. Emily was given advice on allergen avoidance, and how to recognize deteriorating asthma. She also agreed to keep a peak flow diary for one month.

At her review one month later, Emily's peak flow rate was no better, and her diary showed large variations in peak flow recordings, the lowest reading being 180 litres per minute. Emily promised that she had been taking her medication regularly, and there were no problems with her inhaler technique. In view of these findings, the nurse decided to do a spirometry test, and was surprised to find that Emily's lung function was extremely poor, with an FEV1 of only 52 % of predicted. After discussion with the GP, it was decided to give Emily a course of oral corticosteroids, and it was arranged to test her lung function again after that.

Despite being on 30 mg of prednisolone daily for one week, Emily's lung function had not improved significantly. At this stage the nurse started to wonder if Emily did indeed have asthma, or whether there was some other underlying cause for her symptoms. She arranged to meet with Emily and her mother to discuss the problem, and to try to find out more information about Emily's past medical history, and also to look into the family history. It was discovered that Emily's paternal grandmother had died at an early age from some sort of lung problem, but Emily's mother did not know the exact cause of death. Further questioning revealed that Emily's father and uncle both had asthma, and needed frequent hospital admissions. However, as there had been no family contact for the last ten years, she did not know if Emily's father was continuing to have problems with his chest.

Following this discussion, it was decided to check if Emily had alpha-1 antitrypsin deficiency, inherited from her father's side of the family, and a blood test was arranged. The test proved positive, and Emily was referred to a consultant for further advice on management.

Figure 9.3. Emily's story

Clinical Features

You can start your initial assessment of the patient just by simple observation. A patient who is being carried, or wheeled in, is likely to be worse than the patient who walks in unaided. The patient may appear cyanosed or pale, and may be anxious and/or distressed. Check if the patient is able to complete a sentence without taking a breath. All these features can be observed without using any technical equipment or objective measurements.

Once you have made a mental note of the above, move on to the clinical features. These include cough, breathlessness and wheeze in varying degrees, depending on the severity of the attack. Look also for intercostal or subcostal recession. This is when the skin between and under the ribs seems to be sucked in. You may feel you have the necessary knowledge and expertise to do a clinical examination and listen to the patient's chest. Although this may give useful additional information, it is not always necessary in the initial stages of managing the patient with acute asthma.

Objective Measurements

It is important to try to obtain some objective measurements before commencing any drug treatment. This is both to assess the severity of the attack and to measure any response to treatment. The following should be recorded in adults and children over the age of five years.

- Peak expiratory flow rate (PEFR)
- Pulse
- Respirations
- Oxygen saturation (if available)

The peak flow rate should be compared to the patient's previous best peak flow if this is known. If it is not known, then it should be compared to the predicted value for their age, height and sex. In children under the age of five years, peak flow measurements are not terribly reliable so are generally not recorded.

- A reading of between 50 % and 75 % of previous best or predicted indicates a mild or moderate attack.
- A reading of 33–50 % of previous best or predicted indicates an acute severe attack.
- A reading of less than 33 % of previous best or predicted is a sign of a life-threatening attack.

The severity of the attack can be classified according to peak flow rate, and pulse and respiration rate as shown in Table 9.2.

A pulse oximeter is a relatively cheap and easy way to assess oxygen saturations and all accident and emergency departments and most GP surgeries will have access to one. Oxygen saturations of less than 92 % indicate life-threatening asthma. Arterial

Table 9.2. Features of acute severe and life-threatening asthma

Acute severe asthma	Life-threatening asthma
• PEFR 33–50 % of best or predicted • Respirations >25 breaths/min • Pulse >110 beats/min • Unable to complete sentences in one breath	• PEFR <33 % of best or predicted • SpO$_2$ <92 % • Bradycardia • Dysrhythmia • Hypotension • Silent chest • Cyanosis • Feeble respiratory effort • Exhaustion • Confusion • Coma

blood gas measurement and chest X-ray may be indicated if the patient has life-threatening asthma, but this will only usually be available in an acute hospital setting.

It is very important to be aware that not all patients with life-threatening asthma will be distressed. Children particularly may appear quiet, calm and perhaps not even breathless. This tends to happen later on in an attack when they become tired and generally give up fighting for breath. If you put a stethoscope on their chest, there may be no sound of air moving through the airways at all. This is known as a 'silent chest' and is a very dangerous sign which could be a prelude to respiratory failure.

The features of acute severe and life-threatening asthma in adults and children are summarized in Table 9.2.

> Patients with features of acute severe, or life-threatening asthma should be admitted to hospital urgently.

When you have done your assessment, you can make a decision on the best management for the patient. You may decide that the patient needs to be admitted to hospital, and ambulance transfer should be arranged as soon as possible. However, treatment should be started immediately, and can also be continued while the patient is being transported to hospital. Many nurses now work autonomously in situations where there is no medical supervision or support. If you are in this position, it is important that guidelines or protocols are in place to protect both you and your patients. Patient group directions for the administration of drugs may need to be developed, in this case a short-acting bronchodilator, for example salbutamol, and a one-off dose of oral prednisolone. As more nurses become independent prescribers, the use of patient group directions may diminish; however, they are a very useful tool in the management of acute asthma, and allow nurses to commence possibly life-saving treatment. The earlier the treatment is started, particularly in the administration of corticosteroids, the better the outcome.

THE TREATMENT OF ACUTE ASTHMA

An acute asthma attack is an extremely frightening situation, both for the patient and their family or friends. Patients are likely to be distressed and their relatives very anxious, so it is important to try to keep as calm as possible and constantly offer reassurance. Patients will probably find sitting upright more comfortable than lying down and will not appreciate having an arm put around their shoulders. If you feel they need to be comforted, holding their hand is a much better option as this does not restrict their breathing.

OXYGEN

The patient with acute asthma will invariably be hypoxic. Oxygen should therefore be given at a high flow concentration, usually 40–60 %. The aim is to maintain oxygen saturations above 92 %.

DRUG TREATMENT FOR AN ACUTE ATTACK OF ASTHMA

B2 Agonists

Immediate drug management is with a B2 agonist, for example salbutamol or terbu-taline given via an oxygen-driven nebulizer if available. An oxygen flow rate of 6–8 l per minute needs to be achieved to nebulize the drug. If oxygen is either not available or not able to be delivered at the desired flow rate, the drug can be given through an air-driven nebulizer. If neither a nebulizer nor oxygen are available, repeated actuations of a B2 agonist metered dose inhaler can be given through a spacer device.

Corticosteroids

Giving systemic corticosteroids at the earliest opportunity, preferably within 1 h, in an acute asthma attack has been shown to reduce mortality, relapses and subsequent hospital admissions [3]. The usual dose for adults is 40 mg prednisolone, preferably using dissolvable tablets as these have a slightly quicker onset of action. For children aged 2–5 years, the dose is usually 20 mg, and for children aged 5 years and over, the dose is usually 30–40 mg. Children under the age of 2 years should receive 10 mg of soluble prednisolone. Injected corticosteroids have no advantage over oral corticosteroids unless the patient is unconscious or vomiting and therefore unable to swallow tablets. The prednisolone is then carried on daily for at least five days, or until recovery. In the case of small children, under the age of two years, the tablets are usually taken for three days. The course of tablets does not need to be tapered off unless the patient needs to take them for more than three weeks.

Anticholinergics

In life-threatening or acute severe asthma, the addition of the anticholinergic drug ipra-tropium via oxygen-driven nebulizer has been shown to increase bronchodilatation and lead to faster recovery. It can be mixed with the B2 agonist in the same nebulizer for ease of use. Ipratropium is not thought to be beneficial in milder exacerbations of asthma.

Magnesium Sulphate

In recent years, intravenous magnesium sulphate has been increasingly used in the management of acute asthma. It is usually given as a single dose in an infusion over 20 min when the patient is failing to respond to conventional treatment. More research is needed, however, to determine the frequency and/or dosage of magnesium therapy before it becomes more widely used.

Aminophylline

Another option for drug treatment is intravenous aminophylline, but this is usually only used if standard treatment has failed. It should be administered in a slow infusion over 20 min. Care should be taken if the patient is already on oral maintenance treatment with theophylline, as there is the risk of a potential overdose.

Antibiotics

Antibiotics are not routinely prescribed in the management of acute asthma, unless there is an underlying infection.

Sedatives

The use of sedatives should be avoided in acute asthma, unless the patient needs to be ventilated.

ADMISSION TO HOSPITAL

Following emergency treatment, a decision has to be made as to whether to admit the patient to hospital or discharge them home. In a big accident and emergency department, this decision will usually be made by the supervising doctor. However, in these days of advancing nursing practice, increasing numbers of nurses are working at a higher level and are qualified to assess, treat and discharge patients without referral to a doctor. Other nurses working in the community follow protocols and guidelines for the management of acute asthma, and are also able to discharge patients.

Sometimes the decision on whether to admit or not to admit is easy. For example, the patient who has presented with a life-threatening or acute severe attack will definitely need to be admitted. The patient who presents with a mild or moderate attack, however, may be discharged and this is discussed further on in this chapter. Other factors to take into consideration include time of presentation. For example, if the patient presents in the late afternoon or evening, it is probably better to admit them. Previous hospital admissions, and severe attacks should also be taken into account. Social circumstances are also important. If the patient is elderly and lives alone, it

Table 9.3. Criteria for admission to hospital

Admit the patient to hospital if any of the following are present	Other factors to consider
• Life-threatening features • Features of acute severe or life-threatening asthma still present after initial treatment • Patient not responding to treatment • Any episodes of previous near fatal asthma	• Previous hospital admissions • Patient presents in the afternoon or evening • History of previous severe attacks • Doubt over patient's, or carer's, ability to act appropriately in the event of worsening symptoms • Any concern about psycho/social circumstances

may not be advisable to discharge them. It is also important to assess the patient's, or carer's, understanding of their condition. Are they able to act appropriately if their condition worsens? The criteria for admission are summarized in Table 9.3.

Further Management

Following initial treatment, the patient needs constant monitoring. Oxygen saturations should be monitored carefully, with the aim of maintaining oxygen levels at above 92 %. Peak flow rate should be recorded regularly, together with pulse and respiration rates. Skin colour, levels of breathlessness and other symptoms should be observed.

The patient will probably need high dose nebulized bronchodilators at least four hourly, but more often if necessary. Oxygen may also have to be continued to maintain oxygen saturations at above 92 %. Oral predisolone should be given daily, usually in the morning. More often than not, the patient will recover quickly on this regime. However, sometimes things do not go according to plan and the patient may need more aggressive management. Repeated administration of a B2 agonist will be necessary and ipratropium could be included in the nebulized medication. The addition of other drugs may have to be considered, for example, theophylline and magnesium may be used intravenously and some patients may need to be rehydrated and electrolyte imbalance corrected. Care should be taken when using high doses of B2 agonists as they can sometimes cause hypokalaemia.

A chest X-ray may be performed to exclude any other underlying problems such as a pneumothorax, and blood gas analysis carried out to assess levels of hypoxaemia and hypercapnia. If the patient becomes weak and tired, and shows signs of poor respiratory effort, it may be necessary to mechanically ventilate them. Those patients who do not respond to therapy, or need ventilatory support will need to be admitted to a high dependency or intensive care unit.

Discharge

Discharge from hospital should be planned well in advance of the actual discharge date, although in reality this is often quite difficult to achieve. Clinical signs should be stable and peak flow back to normal. Nebulized therapy should be discontinued and the patient well established on inhalers at least 24 h prior to discharge. Advice should be given on what to do in the event of worsening asthma, perhaps giving the patient an 'open door' policy for a specified period of time.

Many patients, particularly those who have a moderate exacerbation, will be discharged from the accident and emergency department, or surgery, following treatment. Before leaving it is important to ensure that the patient understands that they should return if there is any deterioration in their condition. It is also important to check inhaler technique and make sure that the patient has a supply of their medication at home. If the patient has been given a course of oral corticosteroids, they should be told to take each dose all in one go every morning and to make sure they finish the course. A follow-up appointment should also be given before discharge. If possible try to give all this information in the form of a written management plan.

Follow-up and Review

All patients who have had an acute exacerbation of their asthma should receive a follow-up appointment with their GP or practice nurse as soon as possible after the event, preferably within 48 h. If the patient has been admitted to hospital, it is recommended that they are followed up by a respiratory specialist within 30 days. It is important to try to find out the reason for the exacerbation and discuss with the patient management strategies for any possible future episodes. The reasons for the exacerbation may not always be evident, but often it is possible to identify triggers for the attack. With children, for example, what typically happens is that they have a cold, the weather may be damp or misty and then they go to visit a friend who has a cat or dog. The child may be well able to cope with the first two events, but coming into contact with the animal is the final straw.

It is also important to review the patient's medication and check inhaler technique and concordance with their inhalers. Drug treatment and/or inhaler devices may need to be changed as a result of your assessment. The patient should be provided with a written asthma action plan with agreed actions to be taken in the event of deteriorating asthma. Asthma action plans are discussed in more detail in Chapter 7.

DISCUSSION

Deteriorating asthma is a significant feature which needs urgent attention in order to prevent a possibly life-threatening episode of asthma. In some way it can be seen as a failure of management, either by the patient or by the clinician looking after them. There have been a number of studies published looking into this issue of asthma management, including the earlier study done by the British Thoracic Association [4] in 1982 which showed that over 80 % of asthma deaths could have been prevented. More recent studies [5–7] have found that under-use of inhaled and/or oral steroids, inadequate monitoring and follow up and under-use of management plans had a big part to play in many asthma deaths. In some cases the patients themselves or their carers had underestimated the severity of the final attack and left it too late before seeking medical help. Psychosocial issues also had a big part to play. The majority of asthma deaths occur before the patient even reaches hospital.

Patient education is therefore vital if we are to improve this situation, together with written asthma action plans giving advice on which signs and symptoms to look out for, and what actions to take in the event of worsening asthma.

CLINICAL GOVERNANCE

At all times through your professional working life, it is important to maintain skills and expertise to the standard at which you are working. You should be able to provide lawful, safe and effective care and acknowledge the limits of your competency. With this in mind it is important to attend any available training regularly and to keep abreast of any developments in your particular area of practice. This is particularly important in the emergency situation when treating a patient with acute asthma.

It is vitally important to document everything, including how the patient arrives, your initial assessment and any objective measurements you may have made, and also the treatment given and response to treatment. This may be quite difficult to do if you are working alone, but it should be done as soon as possible after the event while things are still fresh in your mind. If, in the unfortunate event of the case coming before a court of law, you have not kept complete and accurate records, it will be very difficult to defend yourself against possible disciplinary action. Remember: 'if it is not written down, it didn't happen'.

SUMMARY

This chapter has discussed the issues surrounding deteriorating asthma and also described the management of the acute exacerbation. It has highlighted the importance of recognizing deteriorating asthma, as in the majority of cases there are many signs which, if acted upon quickly, could avert an acute asthma attack. It follows that patient education, together with written action plans, are important aspects of asthma management and every opportunity should be taken to ensure that the patient understands their asthma management and knows what to do when things start to go wrong.

In the event of an acute asthma attack, recognition and accurate patient assessment are extremely important aspects of management. The treatment that follows should be prompt and aggressive, with early use of bronchodilators and oral corticosteroids.

Following an acute asthma attack, follow-up and review of the patient is vital to ascertain what went wrong and to try to find out the reasons or triggers for this event. Medications may have to be adjusted, and inhaler technique and concordance with therapy should be checked. This is also the time either to review the patient's action plan, or provide and discuss a new plan if necessary.

Finally, the issues surrounding clinical governance were discussed. It is extremely important, both for you and your patients, that you accurately record everything that happens. Nurses are increasingly being given, and accepting, more responsibility, but remember that this also brings more clinical accountability.

REFERENCES

1. British Thoracic Society/Scottish Intercollegiate Guidelines Network (2005) *British Guideline on the Management of Asthma*, Revised edition. Available at www.brit-thoracic.org.uk/guidelines.html.
2. Adams, R.J., Smith, B.J., Ruffin, R.E. (2000) Factors associated with hospital admissions and repeat emergency department visits for adults with asthma. *Thorax*, **55** (7), 566–73.
3. Rowe, B.H., Spooner, C., Ducharme, F.M. *et al.* (2005) Early emergency department treatment of acute asthma with systemic corticosteroids. *The Cochrane Database of Systematic Reviews*, (Iss. 1). Art. No.: CD002178: DOI: 10.1002/14651858. CD002178.
4. British Thoracic Association (1982) Deaths from asthma in two regions of England. *British Medical Journal*, **285**, 1251–5.
5. Bucknall, C.E., Slack, R., Godley, C.C. *et al.* (1999) Scottish confidential enquiry into asthma deaths (SCIAD), 1994–1996. *Thorax*, **54** (11), 978–84.
6. Burr, M.L., Davies, B.H., Hoare, A. *et al.* (1999) A confidential enquiry into asthma deaths in Wales. *Thorax*, **54** (11), 985–9.
7. Sturdy, P.M., Butland, B.K., Anderson, H.R. *et al.* on behalf of the National Asthma Campaign Mortality and Severe Morbidity Group (2005) Deaths certified as asthma and use of medical services: a national case-control study. *Thorax*, **60**, 909–15.

10   Other Therapies

Key points:

- Most patients with asthma will respond well to conventional asthma treatments.
- There are a small percentage of people with asthma who need more complex treatments, and these patients will be under the care of a respiratory specialist.
- Other treatments include immunosuppressant drugs, subcutaneous bronchodilators and immunotherapy.
- Influenza vaccine is recommended for patients with chronic respiratory disease.
- Pneumococcal vaccine is routinely offered, although the evidence for this is not strong.
- Many people with asthma use complementary medicines, and other alternative therapies but the evidence for their efficacy is limited.

INTRODUCTION

Modern medicines are extremely effective in controlling asthma, especially since the introduction of inhaled steroids and long-acting bronchodilators. However, there are a few asthmatics who, for whatever reason, either do not respond to these drugs or whose asthma is very difficult to control despite being on high doses of oral steroids and other asthma drugs. These patients will probably be under the care of a specialist chest physician who may decide to look at other possible therapies in an effort to control the patient's symptoms. This chapter explores some of the other treatments available for the management of this 'difficult to manage' group of patients, but bear in mind that research is advancing in this field of asthma care and newer, more effective treatments may appear at any minute.

In this chapter, I have aimed to describe the different sorts of treatment currently available, but it is beyond the scope of this book to discuss them in any great detail because of the complexities involved. Any patient who is on this type of treatment will be under the care of a specialist who has the necessary experience and knowledge to carry out complicated drug therapy.

IMMUNOTHERAPY

Immunotherapy, or desensitization, has been available for many years, but because of the risks associated with the procedure, is not used to any great extent. It involves injecting gradually increasing quantities of an allergen extract under the skin, which modifies the immune response. Immunotherapy has been shown to decrease asthma symptoms, and improve bronchial hyperreactivity [1], but these benefits must be considered in relation to the possible adverse effects. Introducing an allergen to a patient leads to a high risk of anaphylaxis and death. If it is done at all, it will be performed in specialist centres and by clinicians who have a lot of experience in this type of treatment.

ANTI-IgE THERAPY

Immunoglobulin E (IgE) is produced when the body comes into contact with an allergen. The IgE then combines with inflammatory receptors on the mast cells, leading to the cascade of events which results in inflammation and smooth muscle constriction. The aim of anti-IgE therapy is to block IgE from initiating this allergic response. The drug in current use is omalizumab, which is a recombinant humanized monoclonal antibody. It works by inhibiting IgE from attaching to mast cells, thereby preventing IgE mediated inflammatory changes. It is given by subcutaneous injection two to four times a month, depending on asthma symptoms. The dose is determined by body weight and levels of IgE present, and is licensed only for children and adults over the age of twelve years. It should only be considered for those patients who have proven consistent allergies to airborne allergens and who have uncontrolled asthma despite being on optimum conventional therapy.

At present there is not enough data to ascertain its safety in pregnancy or in breastfeeding, so the current recommendation is that it should not be used in either of these situations. The most common side effects of omalizumab are headaches and local reactions at the site of injection. Other less common side effects include dizziness, drowsiness, nausea, diarrhoea and postural hypotension.

ALPHA-1 ANTITRYPSIN AUGMENTATION THERAPY

Alpha-1 antitrypsin is a protein present in normal lungs and protects lung tissue from being digested by destructive enzymes. Deficiency of alpha-1 antitrypsin therefore results in gradual destruction of the lung tissue. It is an inherited condition where both parents will carry the gene. Patients may be either totally deficient or have lower levels than normal.

In the United States and Canada, alpha-1 antitrypsin augmentation therapy is available which involves a weekly intravenous infusion of alpha-antitrypsin derived from donated human plasma. However, evidence that this treatment is effective is still very scarce and the UK is still in the experimental stages of this type of therapy.

SUBCUTANEOUS BRONCHODILATORS

The majority of asthma treatment is given by the inhaled route with very good effect. However, some patients, especially those with brittle asthma, do not respond so well to traditional treatment. Long-term continuous infusion of a B2 agonist, usually terbutaline, is sometimes used in patients with brittle asthma with good effect, although it is not known why this seems to work better than giving high dose nebulized B2 agonists.

There are problems with continuous long-term subcutaneous therapy, and many patients are unable to tolerate it for a number of reasons, such as muscle cramps and the development of subcutaneous abscesses. There is also the issue of having a permanent fixture attached to the body, which many people find difficult to cope with.

IMMUNOSUPPRESSANT THERAPY

Immunosuppressant drugs, as their name suggests, suppress the immune system, but their role in the treatment of asthma is to prevent the immune response being triggered, which in some asthmatics is difficult to achieve with traditional therapy. The three drugs most commonly used are methotrexate, cyclosporin and gold. They are also known as steroid sparing agents, meaning that there is less need for long-term oral steroid use. This sort of therapy will be reserved for those patients with severe, uncontrolled asthma, despite being on optimum asthma medication.

Immunosuppressant therapy does carry a number of risks, and therefore should be undertaken in a specialist centre, by clinicians with experience of using these medicines.

Methotrexate

Methotrexate was first used in the 1940s as a treatment for leukaemia, but because of its anti-inflammatory properties, it has been used in the treatment of a number of autoimmune and inflammatory diseases such as rheumatoid arthritis and asthma. How it works, however, is unclear. It does seem to have some effect on the production of leukotrienes, macrophages and monocytes, and also inhibits the release of histamine.

The side effects of methotrexate include liver function abnormalities, abdominal pain, nausea, diarrhoea, headache and rash. Other reported effects are reduced concentration and fatigue. A minority of patients have died as a result of the therapy, usually from conditions such as pneumonia and disseminated varicella zoster.

Cyclosporin

Cyclosporin is a drug that is commonly used in organ transplantation to help prevent rejection of the donated organ. As with methotrexate, it also has an anti-inflammatory effect and inhibits the release of inflammatory mediators from mast cells. Cyclosporin has been shown to block the late asthmatic response, which, if you remember from Chapter 3, usually happens about 6–12 h following the initial exposure to an allergen. It inhibits the production of cytokines, which are one of the agents responsible for the amplified inflammatory reaction in the late asthmatic response.

The side effects of cyclosporin include nephrotoxicity, which is dose-dependent, tremor, hirsutism, hypertension, gum hyperplasia and infections.

Gold

Gold has been used in the treatment of severe asthma for about seventy years, although, as in the other steroid sparing drugs, its mode of action is not completely understood. It appears to decrease neutrophil and macrophage cytosis, and also to inhibit the production of leukotrienes and histamine, which are all important aspects of the inflammatory response. Gold has a variety of side effects including gastro-intestinal upset, pruritic rash, cytopenias, oral ulceration and nephrotic syndrome.

VACCINES

Viral infections are commonly involved in asthma exacerbations, and during influenza epidemics, respiratory morbidity increases together with respiratory mortality in the elderly. Influenza vaccination is automatically offered to all adults over the age of 65 years, and also to those patients over the age of six months who are likely to be more at risk of developing complications, such as patients with chronic respiratory disease, including asthma.

As the influenza virus is constantly changing, the vaccine has to be given every year, and the World Health Organization recommends which strain should be used, depending on the particular viruses that are prevalent at the time.

> Be aware that influenza vaccine is grown in the cavity of chick embryos and therefore should not be given to anyone who has hypersensitivity to eggs.

The other routinely advocated vaccine for asthma is the pneumococcal vaccine. However, the evidence on which this is based is not strong, and more research is needed to determine whether or not it is an effective management strategy. It is currently only recommended for those patients who have severe asthma, requiring frequent courses of systemic corticosteroids. In adulthood, it is generally only given once; however, the Department of Health recently announced it is to be added to the childhood immunization programme and will be offered to all children at two, four and 13 months of age.

COMPLEMENTARY THERAPIES

People turn to complementary medicine for all sorts of reasons. Some because they do not want to use conventional medicines, believing that complementary and alternative therapies work just as well, or in some cases even better. Others use complementary medicines because they feel that their conventional medicine is not helping them, so why not try something else? Some turn to complementary medicines and other therapies out of pure desperation, looking for anything that will help them feel better, and therefore be able to lead a normal life.

It is difficult to ascertain just how many people do use complementary medicines or other forms of treatments for managing their asthma. A recent review of studies, for example, found that the figure varies between 4 and 79 % [2]. A survey conducted by Asthma UK, the British asthma charity found that only 6 % of those questioned used complementary therapies [3]. Is there any evidence that these therapies work? This section of the book will go on to discuss the various options available, with reference to any supporting evidence where available.

HERBAL MEDICINES

It is well known that many drugs have a herbal base, and herbal treatments have been in existence for thousands of years. The majority of herbal medicines used in asthma are of Chinese origin. *Ginkgo biloba*, for example, is a sacred Chinese tree, used in oriental medicine since ancient times to improve brain function and for respiratory ailments. Its therapeutic effects in relation to asthma are associated with its antioxidant and anti-inflammatory properties. Other Chinese herbal medicines include *Ligusticum wallichii* which is Chinese lovage, again because it is thought to have an effect on inflammation.

One of the most popular herbal medicines in Japan, and also used in China, is a blend of two herbal preparations containing ten different herbs. This medicine, called *Tsumura saiboku-to* is claimed to have a steroid sparing effect, and is used in patients with severe steroid dependent asthma. Other substances thought to be of benefit include dried ivy leaf extract and marijuana which is thought to act as a bronchodilator in asthma.

Is there any evidence that any of these, or any other, herbal medicines have any beneficial effect on asthma? Many studies have been published claiming positive results from using herbal medicines; however, there were many flaws in the way the studies were conducted. The studies were uncontrolled or not blinded, and descriptions of randomization and dropout rates were absent. In the absence of reliable evidence therefore, it is not possible to say whether herbal medicines are of any benefit. A systematic review of 17 randomized clinical trials on the use of herbal medicines in the treatment of asthma, concluded that because of significant methodological flaws, and lack of standardized quality, herbal medicines are of uncertain value in the treatment of asthma [4].

There is a generalized thought among members of the public that herbal medicines are safe and free from side effects. However, none of the drugs described in this section of the book are free from adverse effects. *Ginkgo biloba*, for example, is considered as one of the safest herbal medicines in the world, and yet the side effects include headaches, nausea and convulsions. It also has potential interactions with other drug treatments such as anticoagulant and antiplatelet medicines.

HOMEOPATHY

Homeopathy, from the Greek *homeo*, meaning similar, and *pathos*, meaning suffering, is a system of alternative medicine based on treating 'like with like'. It works on the premise of giving remedies that will produce the same symptoms in a healthy individual, but very much diluted. In asthma, for example, it would mean giving the patient a homeopathic dilution of the allergen implicated in their asthma. The effect of this treatment is thought to be enhanced with vigorous shaking of the medicine. Other aspects of homeopathy include treating the 'whole' person, which is in fact a holistic approach, advocated in the way in which we, as nurses, treat patients in the conventional manner.

There are several controversies about the use of homeopathy which make it difficult to recommend it. Practitioners say that by diluting the medicine, it is being made more powerful, which is obviously inconsistent with the laws of chemistry. In some instances, the substance is so dilute, there is no active ingredient in it at all. Secondly, although many studies do claim that there have been improvements in lung function and symptom control, it is not clear whether the medicine was responsible for this, or the individualized, personal care that patients received. One review [5], concluded that there is not enough evidence to reliably assess the possible role of homeopathy in the treatment of asthma, and the BTS Guideline [6] advises that further research is required before it can be recommended as a treatment for asthma.

ACUPUNCTURE

Acupuncture is a method of treating asthma by introducing very fine needles into certain points of the body. It is thought to act by blocking the action of the parasympathetic nervous system, and to enhance the action of the sympathetic nervous system. If you remember from Chapter 2, these two systems are responsible for constricting and relaxing bronchial smooth muscle. Acupuncture is also thought to decrease inflammation in the airways, thereby reducing the allergic response to allergens.

Similar to the studies on herbal medicines and homeopathy, studies on the effectiveness of acupuncture have shown some benefit, but the studies are flawed and can not therefore be conclusive as to whether acupuncture works or not.

RELAXATION

We know that asthma, and breathing problems in general, can be exacerbated by stress and anxiety, so it stands to reason that any therapy that involves relaxation and anxiety relieving techniques should be helpful to a patient with asthma. However, as in other forms of complementary therapy, the studies that have been done are not conclusive because of poor randomization methods and statistical control.

HYPNOSIS

Studies of hypnosis in patients with asthma have shown some benefits; however, the studies done were poorly controlled and therefore not reliable. A critical review of asthma and hypnosis concluded that the greatest benefits were in those patients who were more susceptible to this form of therapy [7]. More properly controlled studies are necessary before this treatment can be recommended.

BREATHING EXERCISES AND YOGA

There is a lot of anecdotal evidence about the benefits of breathing exercises and asthma. One method particularly, called the Buteyko method, has received considerable attention, and many patients will say they have benefited from it. Other breathing exercises include a technique called pranayama, which is used in yoga and again, many people will say they find this of benefit. However, yoga and breathing techniques in general have not been proven to have any beneficial effect on asthma symptoms per se, but quality of life measures have shown improvement in some studies as shown in a Cochrane Database review [8]. Much more research is needed on this type of treatment to find out if there are any sustainable benefits from breathing exercises for asthma.

THE BUTEYKO BREATHING METHOD

This method of treating asthma was developed by Professor Konstantin Buteyko as a drug-free complementary therapy for controlling the symptoms of asthma. It involves very specific breathing exercises, together with some dietary and lifestyle modifications. Professor Buteyko bases his theory on the belief that patients with asthma chronically overbreathe, thereby depleting the body of carbon dioxide. By regulating the breathing, together with relaxation methods, asthma symptoms are reduced, and there is less need for rescue medication.

What is the evidence though, for this therapy, and does it work? One fairly recent study found improvements in symptom control, and use of reliever medication, but no difference in exacerbation rate or ability to reduce the dose of inhaled steroid [9]. A review of only four published clinical trials concluded that further research is needed to establish whether the Buteyko Breathing Method is effective and if so, how it may work [10].

FAMILY THERAPY

Psychosocial and emotional factors are well known to affect asthma control, and these issues are recognized as being a risk factor for fatal asthma. Some treatment programmes have been developed aimed at improving relationships in the families of children with severe asthma. There have only been two randomized controlled trials in this area, and these were published many years ago. One study showed improvement in peak flow rate and daytime wheeze [11], and the other showed improvement in symptoms and functionally impaired days [12]. More up-to-date research into this field is needed, however, the British Thoracic Society [6], in its Guideline does state that there may be a role for family therapy as an adjunct to pharmacological treatment.

At the present time, despite there being very little evidence to support complementary and alternative therapies in the treatment of asthma, many people are attracted to this form of treatment. For some, it may be because they find these healthcare alternatives to be more in keeping with their own beliefs and philosophies about life in general. The main problem with the current evidence is that most of the published studies are not reliable enough to be able to make any firm recommendations. As health professionals, perhaps we should remain open-minded about this aspect of healthcare, respecting our patients' views and waiting until there is enough robust evidence before finally making up our minds.

DIETARY MANIPULATION

There has been a lot of speculation in recent years about the causes for the increase in asthma prevalence, and diet has been suggested as one possible reason. With our more affluent society, and easier availability of fast foods, there has been a decrease in the intake of fresh fruit, which contain antioxidants, and an increase in the consumption of fatty foods. Scientists have been aware for some time that eating more polyunsaturated fatty acids, as found in oily fish and fish oils, decreases the production of inflammatory mediators.

This has led to studies investigating whether dietary manipulation can affect asthma control, particularly supplementing the diet with vitamins C and E, and fish oil. However, there is no conclusive evidence supporting the hypothesis that altering the diet will have any effect on asthma symptoms. Two studies investigating the addition of vitamins C and E and magnesium to the diet found that there was no difference in outcomes to those in the placebo group [13, 14].

It is recommended, however, that weight reduction in obese people may help to improve asthma control.

SUMMARY

In addition to the normal, conventional treatments for asthma, a variety of other therapies exist, but these are more often used for patients whose asthma is difficult to control despite being on maximum traditional therapy. The management of these patients is complex, and there may well be other contributing factors. They will usually be under the care of a specialist with experience of looking after patients with more complicated needs.

Alternative, or complementary treatments are used by patients for various reasons, either because of health beliefs, or because they do not feel their asthma is being controlled on conventional medications and are looking for relief from other sources. The evidence for these therapies is not very strong, mainly because of unreliable research methods. However, large numbers of people do use complementary and alternative methods of treatment, and their beliefs should be respected. This is an area where trust, and open and frank discussions should take place between the patient and the healthcare professional looking after them.

REFERENCES

1. Abramson, M.J., Puy, R.M., Weiner, J.M. (2003) Allergen immunotherapy for asthma. *Cochrane Database of Systematic Reviews* (Issue 4), Art.No. CD001186. DOI:a0.1002/ 14651858.
2. Slader, C.A., Reddel, H.K., Jenkins, C.R. *et al.* (2006) Complementary and alternative medicine use in asthma: who is using what? *Respirology*, **11** (4), 373–87.
3. Partridge, M.R., Dockrell, M., Smith, N.M. (2003) The use of complementary medicines by those with asthma. *Respiratory Medicine*, **97** (4), 436–8.
4. Huntley, A., Ernst, E. (2000) Herbal medicines for asthma: a systematic review. *Thorax*, **55**, 925–9.
5. McCarney, R.W., Lasserson, T.J., Linde, K., Brinkhaus, B. (2004) An overview of two Cochrane systematic reviews of complentary treatments for chronic asthma: acupuncture and homeopathy. *Respiratory Medicine*, **98** (8), 687–96.
6. British Thoracic Society/Scottish Intercollegiate Guidelines Network (2005) *British Guideline on the Management of Asthma*, Revised edition. Available at www.brit-thoracic.org.uk/guidelines.html.
7. Hackman, R.M., Stern, J.S., Gershwin, M.E. (2000) Hypnosis and asthma: a critical review. *Journal of Asthma*, **37** (1), 1–15.
8. Holloway, E., Ram, F.S. (2004) Breathing exercises for asthma. *Cochrane Database Review*, (1), CD)001277.
9. Cooper, S., Oborne, J., Newton, S. *et al.* (2003) Effect of two breathing exercises (Buteyko and pranayama) in asthma: a randomised controlled trial. *Thorax*, **58** (8), 674–9.
10. Bruton, A., Lewith, G.T. (2005) The Buteyko breathing method for asthma: a review. *Complementary Therapies Medicine*, **13** (1), 41–6.
11. Lask, B., Matthew, D. (1979) Childhood asthma. A controlled trial of family psychotherapy. *Archives of Disease in Childhood*, **54** (2), 116–9.
12. Gustafsson, P.A., Kjellman, N.-I. (1986) Family therapy in the treatment of severe childhood asthma. *Journal of Psychosomatic Research*, **30** (3), 369–74.
13. Pearson, P.J., Lewis, S.A., Britton, J., Fogarty, A. (2004) Vitamin E supplements in asthma: a parallel group randomised placebo controlled trial. *Thorax*, **59** (8), 652–6.
14. Fogarty, A., Lewis, S.A., Scrivener, S.L. *et al.* (2003) Oral magnesium and vitamin C supplements in asthma: a parallel group randomised placebo controlled trial. *Clinical and Experimental Allergy*, **33** (10), 1355–9.

11 Structure of Care

Key points:

- The patient with asthma will come into contact with many different health professionals.
- Good liaison and teamwork is essential to ensure the best possible care for asthmatic patients.
- The majority of healthcare takes place in primary care.
- It is important to maintain a practice register of asthma patients.
- All patients with asthma should be reviewed at least once a year, but this may be more often depending on the severity of the asthma and any other issues that may impinge on control.
- Children with asthma need to be reviewed more often.
- The review of the patient needs to be structured and consistent.
- In many practices the practice nurse is responsible for running asthma clinics and is responsible for much of the care that asthmatic patients receive.
- Other health professionals, such as district nurses and health visitors can play a key role in the management of the patient with asthma.
- Many schoolchildren have asthma; therefore it is important that school staff are aware of the asthmatic children in their care and know how to cope with an acute episode of asthma.
- Teachers do not have a legal duty to administer medications to children, but are required by law to maintain the health and safety of children in their care.
- Many schools have developed a school asthma policy in conjunction with the healthcare community.

INTRODUCTION

Whatever your particular area of healthcare, you are likely to come across someone with asthma at some time during your working life. For example, you may be a district nurse, looking after a patient with leg ulcers, or a health visitor visiting a new mother and her baby. These patients may also have asthma, and your input, however limited, may make a big difference to their asthma care and management. In addition to this, patients with asthma will come into contact with many different members of the healthcare team, in different settings and in different circumstances. For example, the responsibility of the day-to-day management of their asthma will rest with the GP and the practice team, but should a hospital admission be necessary, they will come into contact with a whole new set of healthcare professionals. Other situations where asthma may be a concern include nursing homes, schools and in the community. Occasionally, non-healthcare professionals are involved in this process. This chapter aims to discuss the different aspects of patient care in other settings, and the roles of the people involved.

ASTHMA IN GENERAL PRACTICE

In previous chapters we have discussed the diagnosis, pharmacological, and nonpharmacological, management of the patient with asthma. This section goes on to identify ways of achieving good asthma management, concentrating on the structure of care and review. The majority of asthma patients are managed in primary care and many GP practices produce their own protocols, or guidelines based on the British Thoracic Society (BTS) Asthma Guideline [1]. Added to this, the Quality and Outcomes Framework outlined in the General Medical Services Contract described further on in this chapter, details outcome measures that most practices will strive to achieve.

PRACTICE ASTHMA PROTOCOL

A clear, easy-to-follow asthma management protocol is essential for effective, consistent delivery of care. The protocol should be developed and agreed by all members of the primary healthcare team. It should identify the roles and responsibilities of each member of the practice team, and outline procedures to follow for the diagnosis, follow-up and referral for patients with asthma.

PRACTICE REGISTER OF PATIENTS WITH ASTHMA

In order to be proactive, and plan and effectively deliver care to any patient group, it is important to know the scale of the problem. Active disease registers are therefore vital to plan ahead and direct resources to where they are most needed. The majority of practices now have an asthma register, which is kept up to date to conform to the quality and outcomes framework mentioned previously. An asthma register is also useful in enabling patient reviews in a structured manner.

Since the introduction of the Quality and Outcomes Framework, the majority of GP practices will now have an asthma register. However, if you are working in general practice and are in the unfortunate situation of not having a register, and wonder 'Where on earth do I start in compiling one?', the following pointers might help:

- Check repeat prescriptions for inhaled steroids and bronchodilators.
- Check prescriptions for courses of oral steroids and antibiotics for chest infections.
- Look at hospital admissions and accident and emergency attendances.
- Ask other team members about known patients.

When looking at repeat prescriptions, it is important to be able to differentiate between prescriptions for asthma and COPD, so you will need to check the patient's records to confirm the diagnosis. Where this is still unclear, you may need to call patients in for a review of their diagnosis. It is also useful to keep separate registers of patients with current symptoms, and those who have had asthma in the past but are no longer being treated.

As you can imagine, compiling an asthma register from scratch can be quite a laborious process, and will take some time. However, once a register is established, it is easy to keep it up to date as long as all members of the primary healthcare team are aware of it and know how to access it. Quite often, in many practices, it is the responsibility of one person within the team to maintain it, and ensure that it is current and accurate.

THE GENERAL MEDICAL SERVICES CONTRACT

The General Medical Services Contract [2] was introduced in 2003. One of the components of the new contract is the Quality and Outcomes Framework (QOF) which aims to reward General Practitioners for delivering certain services. The QOF measures achievement against a range of evidence-based indicators, with points being awarded for reaching certain targets. Payments are calculated from the numbers of points achieved. There are four domains within the framework:

- the clinical domain
- the organizational domain
- the patient experience domain
- the additional services domain

The clinical domain contains 76 indicators in 11 areas, mainly in chronic disease management such as asthma, coronary heart disease and COPD. Each disease area has a list of clinical indicators with points awarded for achievement of each target. Table 11.1 lists the clinical indicators for asthma and the numbers of points awarded.

STRUCTURED REVIEW

Every asthmatic patient should be offered the opportunity for a review of their asthma at regular intervals. All patients should receive at least one review per year; however, the frequency of the reviews will depend on the severity of the asthma and any other issues that may impinge on asthma control, such as psychosocial factors. Patients who are receiving high-dose inhaled steroids, those who frequently attend for emergency treatment and children with asthma, will probably need to be seen more often. The use of computers in general practice has made it much easier to be able to target those patients who need more regular review.

Proactive, structured review has been shown to be more effective at reducing symptoms and exacerbations than opportunistic or unscheduled reviews. With this in mind, designated asthma clinics are the best way to provide effective, patient-centred

Table 11.1. Quality and outcomes framework: Clinical indicators for asthma

Clinical indicator	Points awarded
1. The practice can produce a register of patients with asthma, excluding patients with asthma who have been prescribed no asthma-related drugs in the last twelve months.	7
2. The percentage of patients aged eight and over diagnosed as having asthma from 1 April 2003 where the diagnosis has been confirmed by spirometry or peak flow measurement.	15
3. The percentage of patients with asthma between the ages of 14 and 19 in whom there is a record of smoking status in the previous 15 months.	6
4. The percentage of patients aged 20 and over with asthma whose notes record smoking status in the past 15 months, except those who have never smoked where smoking status should be recorded at least once.	6
5. The percentage of patients with asthma who smoke, and whose notes contain a record that smoking cessation advice or referral to a specialist service, if available, has been offered within the last 15 months.	6
6. The percentage of patients with asthma who have had an asthma review in the last 15 months.	20
7. The percentage of patients aged 16 years and over with asthma who have had influenza immunization in the preceding 1 September to 31 March.	12

asthma care. It should be remembered, however, that not all patients will wish to attend for review of their asthma and you may need to be more resourceful in this respect. Telephone consultations, for example, have been shown to be an effective management tool in some areas. Another consideration is to run asthma clinics either early in the morning, or in the evening, to make access easier for people who do not want to take time off work.

Sometimes, even when you feel you are doing everything possible to make clinics more available, there are those patients who simply will not attend for a review. It may be possible to do ad hoc reviews if they attend for another reason, for example the teenager who attends for contraceptive advice. It does not take long to check peak flow or inhaler technique while they are in the surgery. It may be the only chance you get!

When dealing with consistent nonattenders, don't forget the other members of the primary healthcare team. District nurses, health visitors and school nurses, for example, may be able to help with these patients. Good liaison between all healthcare professionals is vital to ensure that the patient with asthma receives the best possible care, and the roles of other members of the team are discussed further on in this chapter.

The issues that need to be covered in a review will depend on the patient and whether they have had any exacerbations, hospital admissions, or accident and emergency attendances. The points covered in the QOF indicators will also have to be recorded. However, there are two basic aspects that must be checked at every review. These are:

• inhaler technique
• concordance with medication

If inhaler technique is less than perfect you may be able to correct it, but a change of device may be necessary. Do not assume because a patient was able to use their device a year ago, the same applies now. Similarly, with concordance with medication, if the patient is not taking their medication regularly as prescribed, you need to find out the reasons why. It may be something simple like forgetting it, or they do not like the taste of their inhaler. In both of these examples, the solution is fairly easy. Some advice on ways to remember their medication and possibly changing the inhaler to something that suits them better will get over this issue.

However, occasionally, the reasons are much more complex involving steroid phobia or perhaps psychological issues. These problems will take much more time and patience to deal with and are discussed in more detail in Chapter 8.

You will need to be able to record objective measurements to be able to monitor the patient's condition. What measurements you record will depend on the available equipment, and skills and knowledge of the person conducting the review. At the very least peak flow rate should be recorded, but you may wish to do spirometry which will provide more information about the patient's lung function. Some patients with asthma keep a diary recording peak flows and symptoms, and it would be a good idea to ask them to bring the diary with them to the review session.

In addition to this, there are certain questions that should be asked to elicit whether the patient's asthma is under control. It is always surprising what asthma patients will put up with and what they see as normal. If you just ask them how they are, they will probably say they are alright. But if you ask open questions like 'How often do you wake at night?' you may well get another answer. To ensure consistency, and to be able to obtain the most useful information as to whether the patient's asthma is under control, the Royal College of Physicians [3] identified three specific questions that should be asked at every review. These are itemized in Figure 11.1.

Other useful tools for monitoring morbidity are the Tayside Stamp [4] or the Jones Morbidity Index [5]. You may, however, want to develop your own tool.

IN THE LAST WEEK/MONTH		
	YES	NO
Have you had difficulty sleeping because of your asthma symptoms (including cough)?		
Have you had your usual asthma symptoms during the day (cough, wheeze, chest tightness or breathlessness)?		
Has your asthma interfered with your usual activities (e.g. housework, work, school etc.)?		

Figure 11.1. Royal College of Physicians' three questions.

DATE:		DAYS OFF/LAST MONTH:
NIGHT-TIME SCORE:	DAY-TIME SCORE:	ACTIVITY SCORE:
ACTUAL PEFR:	COMPLIANCE:	INHALER TECHNIQUE:
% PREDICTED OR BEST:	OTHER EVENTS:	

Figure 11.2. Tayside Asthma Stamp.

THE TAYSIDE ASTHMA STAMP

The Tayside Asthma Stamp [4] acts as an aide memoire for the important aspects of asthma control. It was developed to make asthma consultations more structured, and to assist in the monitoring of the disease. It uses a scoring system to assess asthma control, and can be quickly filled in by the nurse or doctor running the asthma clinic. The Stamp is illustrated in Figure 11.2.

This monitoring tool uses a simple scoring system to assess whether the patient's asthma is under control. The patient is asked the following questions and the score is entered into the relevant box.

Night-time Score

How many nights in the last month have you had difficulty sleeping because of your asthma symptoms (including cough)?

  1 = 1 or 2 × monthly
  2 = 1 or 2 × weekly
  3 = most nights

Daytime Score

How many days in the last month have you had your usual asthma symptoms during the day (cough, wheeze, chest tightness, or breathlessness)?

  1 = 1 or 2 × monthly
  2 = 1 or 2 × weekly
  3 = daily

Activity Score

How many days in the last month has your asthma interfered with your usual activities (e.g. housework, work/school, etc.)?

  1 = 1 or 2 × monthly
  2 = 1 or 2 × weekly
  3 = daily

During the past 4 weeks		
	YES	NO
Have you been in a wheezy or asthmatic condition at least once per week?		
Have you had time off work or school because of your asthma?		
Have you suffered from attacks of wheezing during the night?		

Figure 11.3. Jones Morbidity Index.

Other Events

This section can include reliever use, and date of next review.

THE JONES MORBIDITY INDEX

The Jones Morbidity Index [5] also uses a scoring system to assess asthma control. The patient is again asked three questions as outlined in Figure 11.3, and the answers are scored.

Scoring System

'No' to all questions = low morbidity
One 'yes' = medium morbidity
Two or three 'yes' answers = high morbidity

In this scenario, those patients who have low morbidity do not need any further asthma intervention for another year. Those patients who have medium morbidity require a doctor or nurse appointment to assess the need for further management and those patients who have high morbidity require a full clinic assessment and appropriate follow-up.

RECORD-KEEPING

Accurate record-keeping is vitally important, both for the safe and effective management of the patient, but also to protect yourself. The aim should be for all members of the healthcare team to agree on what information is to be recorded, how it is to be recorded and where the records should be kept. This ensures that continuity of care is not compromised, and that there is effective communication between all team members. In today's 'paperless' National Health Service, most records will be computerized; however, depending on practice protocols, written records may also be kept.

ASTHMA ACTION PLANS

Another part of the review process should include checking whether the patient has an asthma action plan. As discussed in Chapter 7, action plans have been shown to reduce morbidity and improve health outcomes. Each plan should be tailored to the individual, and will need updating to reflect changes in medication, recent exacerbations or patient circumstances. The review appointment gives a good opportunity to ensure that the patient understands their action plan and knows what to do when things start to go wrong.

THE ROLE OF THE PRACTICE NURSE

In general practice, much of the work related to asthma management has been delegated to practice nurses and nurse practitioners. Several studies have shown that nurse run asthma clinics are both cost-effective and a reliable method of delivering patient care, leading to reduced morbidity and improved patient understanding of their condition [6,7]. Depending on qualifications and training, the role will vary as to how much input the nurse will have. At the most basic level, this may be teaching and checking inhaler technique, and recording peak flow measurements. At the other end of the scale, many practice nurses now run asthma clinics and are able to diagnose and manage the condition independently, and with the advent of nurse prescribing, this role has been further enhanced.

If you are in this position, it is important to set boundaries for yourself and ensure that your knowledge base and qualifications are relevant to the level of care you are giving. Remember, you have professional and personal accountability to maintain standards of care, and always act in such a manner that patient safety is not compromised. Working to protocols is the best way of ensuring that both you and your patients are protected from unsafe practices.

AUDIT AND OUTCOME MEASURES

We shall assume you are now running asthma clinics and you feel these clinics are effective and making a difference to asthma care. How do you know this? In order to ensure that the care you are giving is effective, and to plan future strategies, it is important to build some sort of evaluation procedure into your practice. There are various outcome measures that can be employed and what you use will depend on practice protocols and local needs and objectives. You will already probably be recording the outcomes listed in the Quality and Outcomes Framework, but there are other measures you may wish to use. Some general ideas are given below:

- numbers of patients on the asthma register;
- percentage of patients who have had an annual review;
- percentage of patients who have had their inhaler technique checked within the last year;
- numbers of patients presenting for emergency treatment;
- numbers of patients receiving frequent courses of oral steroids;

- numbers of hospital admissions for acute exacerbations;
- percentage of patients who have had lung function testing within the last year (peak flow or spirometry);
- percentage of patients who have an asthma action plan;
- percentage of patients on step 3 or above of the guideline;
- numbers of patients who have been referred to secondary services.

ASTHMA IN OTHER SETTINGS

As previously discussed, the majority of asthma care and management is centred around general practice, and the general practice team of GPs and practice nurses. However, other members of the primary healthcare team also have a part to play, and the rest of this chapter explores these different roles and the contributions they can make to caring for the patient with asthma.

THE ROLE OF THE DISTRICT NURSE

The district nursing team play an important role in the care of patients in the community, and come into contact with a large variety of patients with many different conditions. For example, you may be caring for a patient who has had a stroke, or been discharged from hospital following surgery. There is a possibility that these patients may also have asthma. Even if you are not directly involved in the management of asthma, or perhaps feel that your knowledge about asthma is insufficient to make any big impact, there is usually something you can do that may make a big difference to the patient.

In many cases, you may be the only member of the healthcare team that actually sees the patient in their own home. Education about issues such as healthy lifestyles, allergen avoidance and stopping smoking does not need expert knowledge. You may find that the patient sleeps with the dog or the cat, or lives in a damp caravan, for example. There are some things you will not be able to change, but if the patient's doctor is more aware of any particular problems, the easier it will be for them to manage their asthma.

Checking patient's inhaler technique and concordance with medication regimes are also extremely important. If you are at all unsure or concerned that a patient may not be using their inhalers properly, the GP, or more likely, the practice nurse should be informed so that appropriate measures can be taken.

If you have a special interest in asthma, you may want to play a bigger role in the management of the asthmatic patient. Those patients who are unable to get to the asthma clinic, for example, could be reviewed at home, following the same format as used in the surgery. You may not be able to carry a spirometer around with you (although there are small portable spirometers available), but a peak flow meter is cheap and fits easily into a bag. The patient's GP will also probably be appreciative as it will increase his QOF target points!

THE ROLE OF THE HEALTH VISITOR

Health visitors have a great involvement with children from infancy until they start school. Bearing in mind that the highest proportion of patients with asthma are children, the chances are that health visitors will have a high percentage of asthmatic children on their caseload. Because of their continuing contact with parents and families from birth until the child starts school, health visitors are in an ideal position to be able to give advice and education to families with asthmatic children. The type of advice and education given will depend to a large extent on levels of knowledge and expertise. Some health visitors will be more knowledgeable about asthma and have more expertise than others. They may be able to deliver more in-depth care, such as ensuring the child is on optimum medication as well as being able to educate the parents about the disease and its management. For others, knowledge may be a bit more basic, but even with limited expertise, the health visitor can still make a useful contribution.

In particular, because of the association between childhood asthma admissions and smoking, health visitors could be really proactive in educating parents about the relationship between smoking and asthma in childhood. Quite often health visitors will also be in a position to give advice to women when pregnant, as they may still be involved with an older child when the mother becomes pregnant again. Smoking in pregnancy has been shown to be harmful to the unborn baby for many reasons, one of which is an increased risk of having a wheezy baby. If there is already one asthmatic child in the family, it is highly possible that any subsequent children will also be asthmatic.

The use of inhalers can be problematic in the under fives and again the health visitor is ideally placed to give advice on this. If you are at all unsure, at the very least you will be able to alert the GP or practice nurse if you think there is a problem. Advice and education about taking the medications regularly is also important, especially as many parents will be worried about their child taking steroids. Explaining the reasons for using them, together with reassurance about their safety, may make the difference between having a child who is well and one who is constantly in hospital.

ASTHMA IN NURSING AND RESIDENTIAL HOMES

The number of nursing and residential homes has increased dramatically over the last 10–15 years and the majority of residents are likely to be elderly, with multiple pathologies and problems. Depending on the different levels of care needed, some patients will have responsibility for their own medications, and in others it will be taken over by the nursing staff in the home.

For those staff working in care homes, it is important to be aware of the different conditions that the residents may have, and any medications that the patients may be taking. In many homes, a large percentage of staff will be unqualified, with perhaps only one or two qualified nurses on each shift. It is the nurse in charge's responsibility to make sure that all staff working in the home have regular updates and are working to their level of competency. Again, as in primary care, protocols and guidelines are essential to ensure that patients receive optimum care, and to guide those members of staff who are less knowledgeable about medical conditions and their management.

A protocol could be quite simple, but it should include the clinical signs and symptoms to look out for which indicate either uncontrolled, or deteriorating asthma, and what should be done about them. A plan should be in place outlining the action to be taken in the event of a patient having an acute asthma attack, and every member of staff should be aware of this plan.

ASTHMA IN SCHOOLS

Asthma is the most common chronic disease of childhood, therefore it stands to reason that there will be a large percentage of children with asthma in the classroom. In a class of thirty children, for example, four or five are likely to have asthma. This poses huge problems for school staff, who not only have to help asthmatic children to lead a normal school life, and thus achieve their full potential, but also have to cope with any emergency situation that may arise.

Many schools have adopted a schools asthma policy, usually in conjunction with their local healthcare team. The policy should contain information about asthma and its management, and also what to do in the event of a child having an acute asthma attack. Asthma UK, the national asthma charity, has some excellent information packs about setting up a school's asthma policy which are available via their website: www.asthma.org.uk. A register of children with asthma is helpful, so that all school staff are aware of the asthmatic children in their care.

Many pupils with asthma will need to take their inhalers during the course of the school day. Ideally, children should be responsible for their own inhalers, but they may also need supervision. The school policy should therefore state whether children can carry and administer their own medication. Where this is not practicable, inhalers should be labelled and kept in a cupboard or drawer in the classroom and be easily accessible. In the past it was not uncommon for inhalers to be locked in a cupboard, sometimes in the head teacher's office, and children had to find someone to ask for access to their medication.

Fortunately this situation is changing and recent guidelines published by the Department of Health [8] state that all emergency medicines such as asthma inhalers should be readily available to children and not be locked away. However, it is also important that medicines are only available to those for whom they are prescribed. Arrangements should be in place for availability of these inhalers when the children are away from the classroom, for example when playing games or on school trips.

School staff are frequently worried about medicines and their safety, and are often reluctant to take responsibility for administering medicines to children. Teachers do not have a legal duty to administer medication and if they do decide to take on this responsibility, it is completely voluntary. However, school staff do have a duty of care, and schools by law are responsible for the health and safety of children in their care. In view of this, school staff who volunteer to administer medication need support from the head teacher and parents, access to information and training, and reassurance about their legal liability. In its document, *Managing Medicines in Schools and Early Years Settings*, the Department of Health [8] clearly lays down guidelines outlining schools' responsibilities and encourages schools and Local Education Authorities to ensure that they have the appropriate insurance cover.

Role of the School Nurse

Sadly, in many parts of the country, numbers of school nurses seem to be diminishing. However, they do have a big role to play in the way asthma is managed in schools. Many school nurses have been involved in the development of schools' asthma policies, and are responsible for educating teachers and other school staff about asthma. In some areas, school nurses have set up asthma clinics within schools, particularly targeting teenagers, as this age group are less likely to attend for structured clinical reviews, and more likely to attend for emergency treatment for their asthma. The school nurse is also ideally placed to act as a liaison between all the various services involved in the care of school children. For example, if a child is missing a lot of school because of their asthma, the school nurse should be proactive in trying to find out what is happening to the child and alerting the GP as to possible problems. Obviously this should be done with the full cooperation of the parents, because it is important to be able to have a frank and open discussion.

SUMMARY

This chapter has discussed the importance of structured care for patients with asthma and the role of the different healthcare professionals who may be involved with asthmatic patients. Ensuring constant and consistent care right across the healthcare community, leads to a greater chance of better patient outcomes and improved patient satisfaction.

REFERENCES

1. British Thoracic Society/Scottish Intercollegiate Guidelines Network (2005) *British Guideline on the Management of Asthma*, Revised edition. Available at www.brit-thoracic.org.uk/guidelines.html.
2. Department of Health (2003) Quality and Outcomes Framework. www.dh.gov.uk.
3. Royal College of Physicians (1999) *Measuring Clinical Outcome in Asthma: A Patient-Focused Approach*, London.
4. Neville, R.G., Hoskins, G., Clark, R., *et al.* (2001) A standardised recording system to monitor asthma outcomes. *The Asthma Journal*, **6**, 193–6.
5. Jones, K., Cleary, R., Hyland, M. (1999) Predicted value of a simple asthma morbidity index in a general practice population. *British Journal of General Practice*, **49**, 23–6.

6. Hoskins, G., Neville, R.G., Smith, B., Clark, R.A. (1998) The effect of a trained asthma nurse on patient outcomes in General Practice. Presented at the General Practitioners in Asthma Group Conference June 1998, Oxford.
7. Dickinson, J., Hutton, S., Atkins, A., Jones, K. (1997) Reducing asthma morbidity in the community: the effects of a targeted nurse-run asthma clinic in an English General Practice. *Respiratory Medicine*, **91** (10), 634–40.
8. Department of Health (2005) *Department for Education and Skills. Managing Medicines in Schools and Early Years Settings*, London.

12 The Future

Key points:

- The discovery of the ADAM33 gene indicated that genes do have a part to play in the development of asthma.
- The problem with asthma is that it is a very complex disease and it is likely that there are a number of genes responsible for different aspects of it.
- Early life experiences and the environment may contribute to the development of asthma in some people.
- Patients with asthma are more susceptible to viruses, but it is not known whether viral infections cause asthma, or whether being susceptible to asthma predisposes patients to contracting viral infections.
- Asthmatic patients who have low levels of interferon are more likely to develop viral infections.
- It may become possible to modify the way the asthmatic patient responds to contact with allergens.

INTRODUCTION

The publication of the British Thoracic Society's asthma guidelines in the 1990s, provided clinicians with a logical, structured process to follow, which in general improved the treatment of patients with asthma. However, it is evident that we are still not providing optimum management to enable our patients to live their lives free from symptoms and with no acute exacerbations.

Inhaled corticosteroids and bronchodilators are likely to continue to be the mainstay of asthma treatment for the foreseeable future; however, research into the causes of asthma and what role genetics, viruses and the environment play in the way asthma develops, may lead to some interesting developments and new treatments in the future. There are many research opportunities available and this chapter highlights some of the more probable advances we will see over the next ten years. It also discusses the role of nurses, both now and in the near future.

THE ROLE OF GENETICS

Although we have a much better understanding of asthma now than we did 20–30 years ago, there are still many unanswered questions. Perhaps one of the main issues, and where much of the current research is being concentrated, is what role genetics play in asthma. One of the goals of genetic research is to further our knowledge of the pathophysiology of diseases, in the hope that this will lead to more effective treatments. Another goal is to be able to prevent the disease occurring in those individuals identified as being at risk of developing the disease.

The discovery of the ADAM33 gene in 2002 [1] gave a positive indication that genes are implicated in the development of asthma. ADAM33 is a member of the protease subfamily metalloprotease and was identified as a result of mass screening of more than 450 families from the UK and America. Presence of the gene is thought to increase an individual's susceptibility to developing asthma, and it is also thought to contribute to the airway narrowing, and possibly the airway wall remodelling that occurs in severe asthma. A single gene is responsible for the development of some diseases such as cystic fibrosis, but the problem with asthma is that it is a complex multifactorial disorder and ongoing research suggests that there is no single gene, that is totally responsible, and that the ADAM33 gene is only one of a large number of asthma genes.

Trying to identify the genes responsible for susceptibility to complex conditions like asthma is a major challenge, but significant progress has been made over the last five to ten years. Several areas of the genome have been identified where it is probable that genes exist that lead to increased susceptibility to asthma, and other allergic-type diseases. These genes now need to be isolated and each one investigated to establish what role it plays in the development of asthma. Advances in technology mean that research in this area is now much easier, and cheaper to perform, so we may see some interesting developments in the near future.

EARLY LIFE EXPERIENCE AND ENVIRONMENT

As yet, we don't really know what causes asthma, so there is a lot of work being done to try to find out why some people develop asthma and others don't. It is thought that by having a greater understanding of the causes of asthma, it may be possible to identify those children more at risk from developing the disease before any symptoms become apparent. The role of genetics is just one area of research in this particular field. Other researchers are looking at events, either in utero, or in infancy that may contribute to the diagnosis of asthma later on. These events include respiratory infections, or environmental exposure to certain substances such as cigarette smoke and house dust mite. A particular problem at present is that we do not have very much understanding of the development of the respiratory system during the interuterine and immediate postnatal period. This is partly due to the fact that access to blood analysis, or tissue biopsy is extremely limited, but also because lung function testing in the very young is particularly difficult.

There is also a need to understand the factors involved in the development of asthma, and why there can be a relapse, or remission of symptoms sometimes followed by an increase in symptoms at a later stage. Other questions scientists are trying to answer include trying to identify any factors that contribute to the severity of the disease, and whether the progress of the disease can be modified by early life interventions.

The so-called 'hygiene hypothesis' is also likely to be investigated. If you remember from Chapter 3, this theory suggests that by preventing children coming into contact with infectious diseases, we are stopping them developing immunity to bacteria, and therefore increasing their susceptibility to asthma and other common conditions.

The aim of research in this particular area therefore is to try to identify factors either in utero, or in early life that lead to more susceptibility to developing asthma, with a view to modifying these factors and thus preventing the development of asthma in those most at risk.

VIRUSES AND ASTHMA

Viral infections such as the common cold have long been recognized as a major trigger for asthma symptoms, particularly in childhood. It has been estimated that 80–85 % of asthma exacerbations in childhood are caused by respiratory viral infections. In addition, children with asthma seem to have an increased susceptibility to contracting viral conditions. It is also known that viral infections influence the development of immunity and immune responses throughout life. However, the way in which this happens, and its effect on asthma is still not fully understood.

Bronchiolitis in infancy is a common cause of hospital admissions and has been shown to be a risk factor for the development of childhood wheezing and asthma. The leading causes of bronchiolitis are the respiratory syncytial virus (RSV) and rhinovirus (RV). Most of the research into the role of viruses and bronchiolitis to date has concentrated on RSV, but emerging evidence is suggesting that RV may be more of a contributory factor than was originally thought. There is a need for research into this area to try to determine whether severe respiratory viral infections cause asthma, or whether asthma susceptibility predisposes patients to contracting viral infections. It is hoped that by having a greater understanding of the mechanisms of viruses and their role in asthma, it will lead to better prevention and improved interventional therapies.

Another area which is currently being investigated is the role of interferon in respiratory viral infections. Researchers have found that many patients with asthma produce a lower level than normal of interferon [2]. Interferon is a protein with antiviral properties generated by the immune system. Asthmatic patients who have a low level of interferon are more likely to develop respiratory viral infections and thereby suffer more acute attacks of asthma. The lower the level of interferon, the more severe the asthma attack is likely to be. Work is now progressing to try to develop an inhaler which will deliver interferon directly to the lungs, to increase levels of this particular protein, and thereby help to prevent severe asthma attacks.

IMMUNOLOGY AND IMMUNOTHERAPY AND ASTHMA

The understanding of immunology and immunotherapy, and the role they play in asthma has improved considerably over recent years, leading to the identification of new ways to inhibit the development of asthma, and also to modify the way it presents in certain individuals. The recent work that resulted in the development of anti-immunoglobulin E (IgE) therapy for severe asthma has led to more research into the role of IgE, and has also led to the discovery of certain pathways that may be possible to control in order to override the allergic response to allergens. Work is currently being undertaken to investigate the effect this type of immunomodulation will have on the sensitization that occurs in asthma, and how it can affect the progression to clinical disease.

Other researchers are investigating ways of modifying the action of interleukins (IL). These are a group of cytokines which have an effect on the immune system. Three interleukins that are of particular interest in asthma are IL-4, which influence the production of T-cells and mast cells, IL-9 which stimulates the production of mast cells, and IL-10 which inhibits cytokine production. Both mast cells and cytokines play a large part in the inflammatory process in asthma, so if it were possible to alter the way they respond to contact with allergens, the inflammatory response could perhaps be moderated.

BRONCHIAL THERMOPLASTY

A novel nondrug intervention for asthma has recently been generating a lot of interest. Bronchial thermoplasty is carried out using bronchoscopy and is a procedure by which bronchial smooth muscle is targeted by radio waves, to alter its ability to constrict. Early trials, both in the UK and in various other centres around the world, have shown encouraging results, with little or no adverse events. A bigger trial is being planned and we look forward to the results of this, and all the other research currently underway, with interest.

The management of asthma has improved tremendously over the last ten to fifteen years, and we have seen several new drugs, and inhaler devices, come onto the market, which have made a big difference to asthma management, as well as giving patients more choice and flexibility in their care. We look forward with interest to the results of the research that is currently being undertaken into the role of genetics, and all the other issues that are being investigated. The projects that have been highlighted in this chapter are some of the more promising ones, but there is a lot of research being carried out, and a lot more planned for the future.

REFERENCES

1. Van Eerdewegh, P.R., Little, R.D., Dupuis, J. *et al.* (2002) Association of the ADAM33 gene with asthma and bronchial hyperresponsiveness. *Nature*, **418**, 426–30.
2. Contoli, M., Message, S.D., Laza-stanca, V. *et al.* (2006) Role of deficient type 111 interferon-lambda production in asthma exacerbations. *Nature Medicine*, **12** (9), 1023–6.

13 The Role of Nurses in the Management of Asthma

Key points:

- Nurses are increasingly able to practise autonomously in many settings.
- It is important to be clinically competent and to recognize any limitations.
- There are many ways of improving knowledge base and skills, including attending recognized courses and study days, and reading relevant research articles.
- Good interaction with all members of the healthcare team is important to ensure that asthmatic patients are receiving the best possible care.

INTRODUCTION

Over the last ten years, nurses in general have become much more skilled and able to practise autonomously in many different settings. However exciting this may be, it is important to remember that increased autonomy leads to many more responsibilities, and issues surrounding clinical accountability become more significant. Whatever role you are undertaking, you must be fully competent in carrying out that role, and perhaps more importantly, be aware of your limitations, and not allow yourself to be persuaded to carry out procedures that are not within your clinical capability.

AUTONOMY AND RESPONSIBILITIES

The Nursing and Midwifery Council in its Code of Conduct [1] states that:

1.3 'You are personally accountable for your practice. This means that you are answerable for your actions and omissions, regardless of advice or directions from another professional.'

6.2 'To practise competently, you must possess the knowledge, skills and abilities required for lawful, safe and effective practice without direct supervision. You must acknowledge the limits of your professional competence and only undertake practice and accept responsibilities for those activities in which you are competent.'

A lot will depend on your contract of employment, and the role you play within your practice area. Some nurses, for example, are only expected to check patients' inhaler technique and record peak flow measurements. This obviously requires some very basic knowledge and training. Other nurses will be responsible for the total management of patients, right through from diagnosis to monitoring, and treatment of the acute attack, including writing prescriptions.

There are various courses and training programmes around the country and if you are considering taking a greater role in managing patients with asthma, it is strongly recommended that you attend one of these courses. To be able to prescribe, you will also need to attend a recognized, nonmedical prescribing course. Following on from achieving a qualification in asthma management, continuing professional development is crucial to keeping up to date, and maintaining and improving clinical practice. This can be undertaken in a variety of ways. In some areas, forums have been set up for mutual support and sharing of good practice initiatives. It is important to be knowledgeable about new developments and research, so access to peer-reviewed journals is vital, together with the ability to appraise research studies critically. Conferences and study days are also a good way of keeping up to date, although some of them can be quite expensive to attend. You may wish to keep a professional portfolio which identifies your learning needs, and also maps your personal and professional development as you become more confident in managing patients with asthma.

This is quite an exciting time for nurses, the last five years having seen the introduction of nurse consultants and increasing autonomy for nurse practitioners and specialist nurses. This increasing autonomy, however, also means that there will be higher levels of scrutiny, so we must find ways to evaluate our work, and be prepared to change our ways of working to reflect current needs and resources. It is also important to remember that we are part of a team and cannot work in isolation. To provide best possible care for our patients with asthma, we must be able to interact effectively with all members of the healthcare team.

SUMMARY

The role of nurses has changed considerably over the last decade, and there is considerable opportunity for nurses to play a greater part in the management of many chronic diseases, not just asthma. The important message is to make sure you are competent in that role, and not take on any roles or responsibilities for which you have not received the necessary training.

REFERENCE

1. Nursing & Midwifery Council (2002) *Code of Professional Conduct*, NMC, London. www.nmc-uk.org.

Glossary

Adrenaline	A hormone that is released from the adrenal glands during times of stress, leading to increased heart rate, raised blood pressure and widening of the airways.
Airway wall remodelling	Ongoing inflammation that is not controlled can lead to structural changes in the airways, including fibrosis of the airway wall, thickening of the basement membrane and eventually leading to irreversible airway narrowing.
Alpha-1 antitrypsin deficiency	Alpha-1 antitrypsin is a protein that protects the lungs from the destructive effects of certain enzymes. Deficiency of the protein allows enzymes to digest healthy lung tissue. It is an inherited condition.
Alveolus: (pleural alveoli)	The terminal points of the respiratory system, responsible for the exchange of oxygen and carbon dioxide.
Anatomical dead space	The air that remains in the airways and is unavailable for gas exchange.
Anticholinergics	Drugs which block the bronchoconstricting action of the parasympathetic nervous system.
Atopy	The tendency to produce large amounts of immunoglobulin E in response to contact with an allergen
B2 agonists	Bronchodilating drugs which mimic the action of the sympathetic nervous system. They combine with B2 receptors in the bronchial smooth muscle to produce bronchodilatation.
British Thoracic Society Guideline	A guideline produced by the British Thoracic Society in 1993, and updated several times since then. It advocates a stepwise approach to the management of asthma.
Brittle asthma	Asthma that is difficult to control, or sudden severe attacks on a background of apparently well-controlled asthma.

Bronchial hyperreactivity	Also known as airway hyperresponsiveness. This is the tendency of the airways to overreact to contact with allergens, causing airway narrowing and leading to the symptoms of asthma.
Bronchioles	The smaller airways leading into the alveoli.
Bronchus: (pleural bronchi)	The air passage(s) that carry inhaled air from the nose and mouth to the bronchioles. They are divided into main, lobar and segmental bronchi.
Chlorofluorocarbons (CFCs)	A propellant used in some aerosol inhalers, and known to damage the atmosphere.
Cholinergic receptors	Part of the protective response of the parasympathetic nervous system. When stimulated they produce bronchoconstriction.
Concordance	A term to describe a partnership between the patient and the healthcare professional. Nonconcordance could be applied to a patient's use of their drug therapy or to their behaviour, for example not seeking medical help for worsening asthma.
Cor pulmonale	Right-sided heart failure secondary to severe lung disease.
Corticosteroids	Hormones that are produced naturally by the adrenal glands. Synthetically produced corticosteroids are used to reduce the inflammation, and subsequent airway narrowing that occurs in asthma. The corticosteroids can be given in an inhaled form or orally.
Cromones	Drugs which inhibit various inflammatory cells that play a part in the inflammatory process in asthma.
Cytokines	A group of interleukins which are involved in the inflammatory response.
Differential diagnosis	A diagnosis other than asthma, but with similar signs and symptoms.
Dry powder device	An alternative to an aerosol inhaler, which contains the drug in a powder format.
Early response	An early reaction to contact with an allergen. Usually occurs within 5–10 min and lasts about 1–2 h.
Eosinophils	Inflammatory cells implicated in the immune response.
FEV1	Forced expiratory volume in one second. The amount of air that can be forcibly exhaled in one second, starting from a position of full inhalation.
Fibrosis	Scarring of tissue leading to loss of elasticity.
FVC	Forced vital capacity. The total amount of air that can be forcibly exhaled, starting from a position of full inhalation.

Hydrofluorocarbons (HFCs)	A propellant used in newer aerosol inhalers which does not damage the atmosphere.
Immunoglobulin E (IgE)	Produced when the body comes into contact with an allergen. The IgE then goes on to combine with other inflammatory cells, most notably mast cells, leading to a cascade of events resulting in the symptoms of asthma.
Immunosuppressant therapy	Drugs which suppress the immune response. Occasionally used in severe asthma which is resistant to the more conventional forms of treatment.
Immunotherapy	Injecting gradually increasing doses of an allergen extract to modify the immune response.
Interleukins	Numbered 1–33, each one has a different function in the inflammatory response.
Late response	A late reaction to contact with an allergen. Usually occurs 6–12 h following exposure, and is much more difficult to treat than the early response.
Leukotriene receptor antagonists	Drugs which block the production of leukotrienes, an important aspect of the inflammatory response.
Mast cells	Inflammatory cells which are an important part of the immune response.
Mediators	Substances such as histamines and prostaglandins which are released when an atopic individual comes into contact with an allergen. This leads to a cascade of events resulting in inflammation and narrowing of the airways.
Methylxanthines	A group of bronchodilating drugs, usually known as theophyllines.
Mucociliary clearance system	The respiratory system's first line of defence which consists of the mucous glands, goblet cells and cilia.
Nebulizer	A machine which runs off electricity, or can be battery powered. It is used to deliver high doses of inhaled drugs such as bronchodilators. Although commonly known as a nebulizer, the machine is in fact a compressor. The nebulizer component is the small chamber into which the drug is put.
Occupational asthma	Asthma that is caused by the environment in which the affected person works.
Oxygen saturation	The percentage of haemoglobin saturated with oxygen (oxyhaemoglobin).
Peak expiratory flow rate (PEFR)	The rate at which air can be blown out of the lungs with a forced expiration. It is measured in litres per minute.

Physiological dead space	Occurs in diseases such as emphysema where the alveoli are damaged and unable to take part in gas exchange.
Pleura	A continuous serous membrane covering the surface of the lungs and the inner surface of the thoracic cavity.
Primary prophylaxis	Interventions made before there is any evidence of disease to try to prevent its occurrence.
Pulmonary diffusion	The process by which molecules pass from an area of greater concentration to an area of lower concentration. In gas exchange this means that oxygen moves from the alveoli to the capillaries, and carbon dioxide moves from the capillaries to the alveoli.
Pulmonary perfusion	The process by which de-oxygenated blood enters the heart on the right-hand side, and is carried by the pulmonary arteries to the lungs to pick up oxygen and re-enters the heart on the left-hand side.
Radioallergosorbent test (RAST)	A blood test to detect allergies against common antigens.
Reversibility test	A diagnostic test to establish whether there is any reversibility to bronchodilators or oral corticosteroids. A positive result is indicative of a diagnosis of asthma.
Secondary prophylaxis	Interventions made after the onset of disease to try to reduce its impact.
Spacer	A device into which a metered dose inhaler is fired and which holds the drug for a short period of time, thus avoiding the problems of coordination.
Trachea	A muscular tube supported by C-shaped rings of cartilage, and bronchial smooth muscle.

Useful Addresses

Association of Respiratory Nurse Specialists (ARNS), 17, Doughty Street, London, WC1N 2PL
Tel: 0207 269 5793
Website: www.arns.co.uk

Asthma UK, Summit House, 70, Wilson Street, London, EC2A 2DB
Tel: 020 7786 4900
Website: www.asthma.org.uk

British Lung Foundation, 73–75 Goswell Road, London, EC1V 7ER
Tel: 020 7688 5555
Website: www.lunguk.org

British Thoracic Society, 17, Doughty Street, London, WC1N 2PL
Tel: 020 7831 8778
Website: www.brit-thoracic.org

National Respiratory Training Centre, The Athenaeum, 10, Church Street, Warwick, CV34 4AB
Tel: 01926 493313
Website: www.nrtc.org.uk

Index

Complied by Indexing Specialists (UK)